The
Hepatitis C
Sourcebook

HOWARD J. WORMAN, M.D.

D0107766

Contemporary Books

Chicago New York San Francisco Lisbon London Madrid Mexico City
Milan New Delhi San Juan Seoul Singapore Sydney Toronto

Library of Congress Cataloging-in-Publication Data

Worman, Howard J.
    The hepatitis C sourcebook / Howard J. Worman.
        p.   cm.
    Includes bibliographical references and index.
    ISBN 0-7373-0596-7
    1. Hepatitis C—Popular works.   I. Title

    RC848.H425 .W674 2002
    616.3′623—dc21   2001053693

Contemporary Books

A Division of The **McGraw·Hill** Companies

2 3 4 5 6 7 8 9 10 AGM/AGM 1 10 9 8 7 6 5 4 3 2

ISBN 0-7373-0596-7

This book was set in Sabon by Rattray Design
Printed and bound by Quebecor Martinsburg

Cover design by Jeanette Wojtyla
Interior illustrations by Miyake Illustration

McGraw-Hill books are available at special quantity discounts to use as premiums and sales promotions, or for use in corporate training programs. For more information, please write to the Director of Special Sales, Professional Publishing, McGraw-Hill, Two Penn Plaza, New York, NY 10121-2298. Or contact your local bookstore.

This book is printed on acid-free paper.

Dedicated to Terry

Contents

Preface

I HAVE WRITTEN this book from the perspective of both a cell biologist and an internist specializing in liver diseases. As a cell biologist, I am somewhat more attuned to fundamental research and its implications than most practicing physicians. I present what's known about hepatitis C and supported by scientific research and clinical studies. I alert the reader to claims about the disease that are not supported by scientific data. As a liver specialist, I have seen the entire spectrum of patients with hepatitis C, and I understand their concerns. I keep the entire patient in mind, knowing that other life and health matters may be more important than having hepatitis C. Being an internist and not a pediatrician, I focus on adults, not infants or children.

The material in this book is primarily for the layperson. Some health professionals involved in the care of patients with liver disorders may also find it useful. The book's aim is to help the reader develop an overall understanding of hepatitis C, the virus that causes it, what a doctor thinks about when seeing patients with the disease, and what treatments are available now and what's possible for the future. I encourage readers to approach this book with two hopeful thoughts: A diagnosis of hepatitis C is *not* a death sentence and ongoing research will lead to better future treatments for the disease.

This book is *not* a substitute for professional medical care. *Only an experienced physician who knows the complete history and sees the patient can make a diagnosis and offer treatment recommendations.* For readers seeking more information, details about comprehensive sources are provided. I have also included contact information for some legitimate support groups and information organizations for patients with chronic hepatitis C. My book *The Liver Disorders Sourcebook*, published by Contemporary Books, is a more general work on the liver in health and disease.

Several individuals have been helpful in the writing of this book from start to finish. My mother and father, Dora and Louis Worman, put me through college and medical school and provided me with the education that made this work possible. My mentors, Dr. Günter Blobel at Rockefeller University and the late Dr. Fenton Schaffner at Mount Sinai School of Medicine, taught me the basic science and clinical skills necessary to understand hepatitis C, from basic virology to the care of patients. I also would like to thank Edwin Baum for providing important legal advice and Arlene M. Sklar and Louis Worman for help with business matters. My frequent discussions with Dr. Jean-Claude Courvalin at the Institut Jacques Monod in Paris and Dr. Howard P. Reynolds were, as always, very stimulating. Finally, I thank my wife Terry who has always supported me while I spend far too much time in the laboratory, library, and clinic.

1

Viruses and Viral Hepatitis

THE WORD *HEPATITIS* means inflammation of the liver. A number of factors cause hepatitis: alcohol and drugs; toxins; autoimmunity; circulatory problems, such as heart failure (ischemic hepatitis); fatty liver (nonalcoholic steatohepatitis, or NASH); and viruses. Liver inflammation caused by viral infection is called *viral hepatitis*.

Viruses are among the simplest life forms. Like other life forms, viruses reproduce and mutate, or randomly change their genetic material; however, viruses do not have an independent metabolism and can replicate only within cells. Viruses are much smaller than the cells in the human body. They range in size from about 15 to 250 nanometers long. There are a billion nanometers in a meter, which is roughly equal to one yard. About one trillion viruses laid end to end would cover the length of an American football field. For comparison, the human red blood cell, one of the smallest cells in the body, is about thirty times the size of the largest virus. Hepatocytes, the predominant liver cells, are much larger than the viruses that infect them.

Viruses and other life forms (plants, animals, protozoans, yeast, bacteria, and archebacteria) contain genetic material. But whereas the genetic material in most other life forms is deoxyribonucleic acid (DNA), viruses can have either DNA or ribonucleic acid (RNA). The

1

hepatitis C virus, as well as the hepatitis A, D, and E viruses, have RNA as their genetic material; the hepatitis B virus has DNA.

This viral genetic material contains the blueprint for synthesizing various proteins. Some of these proteins are the building blocks of the viral particle. Most viruses have proteins that form the central core or nucleocapsid of the virus, which the RNA or DNA wraps around. Some viruses have a lipid or fatty envelope that fuses with the membrane of the cell they invade. This lipid envelope usually contains specific viral proteins generally referred to as *envelope proteins*. Most viruses also produce proteins that perform essential biochemical functions necessary for their replication. These nonstructural proteins are expressed in the cells that the virus infects and synthesize copies of the virus's RNA or DNA. These nonstructural proteins may be absent from the mature viral particle.

An important property of viruses, as well as of all life forms, is the ability to mutate. Because the genomes of viruses are small and replicate rapidly, their mutation rates are high. Constant mutation allows viruses to escape detection by the host's immune system. For this reason, it is sometimes impossible for the body to clear a viral infection. Mutation also makes it difficult to design drugs against viruses as they can change the viral proteins the drugs target.

Viruses can be thought of as molecular parasites: They use the energy sources, chemical compounds, and protein synthesis machinery of the cells they infect. Viral infection in humans can lead to disease and sometimes death because either the virus itself, or the body's immune response directed against the viral constituents, kills the cells infected with a virus.

When the body is infected with a virus, the immune system usually recognizes the virus as foreign and attempts to eliminate it. The immune system responds in two general ways. One way is a cell-mediated immune response in which specialized cells of the immune system, such as T cells, which recognize cells infected by the virus, are activated. These cells destroy virally infected cells, generally by recognizing viral particles expressed on the cell surface.

The second way the immune system reacts to an infecting virus is by a humoral or antibody-mediated response. In this process, B cells are activated and produce antibodies against the infecting virus.

These antibodies circulate in the blood and recognize mature viral particles as well as proteins expressed in infected cells. The antibodies are generally directed against pieces of viral proteins.

Various methods are used in the laboratory to detect antibodies in the blood against particular proteins. The most common is the enzyme-linked immunosorbent assay (ELISA). This assay takes advantage of the tight binding between an antibody and the protein it recognizes. In the ELISA, a protein is fixed in a plastic dish. Serum, blood containing antibodies but no blood cells, is added to the dish. The dish is then rinsed to remove components not tightly associated with the protein. A second antibody that recognizes the first is added; this antibody sticks to the dish only if the first antibody is present. The dish is then rinsed again. This second antibody is modified chemically so that it can be readily detected by a color change of the solution in the dish. The presence of the second antibody indicates that the first antibody is in the blood and has bound to the protein.

An important property of viruses is *tropism*: the virus's ability to infect a particular type of cell. Viruses that cause hepatitis are referred to as *hepatotropic* because they infect hepatocytes, the major cells of the liver. Hepatotropic viruses can infect other cells besides hepatocytes. Different viruses have different cellular tropisms. For example, the human immunodeficiency virus (HIV) primarily infects certain cells of the immune system, and the rheoviruses that cause diarrhea infect cells of the intestine.

There are five major human viruses that are hepatotropic: hepatitis A, hepatitis B, hepatitis C, hepatitis D (which can only infect people also infected with hepatitis B virus), and hepatitis E. These human hepatitis viruses are very different from one another and cause different types of liver disease. Virologists often classify them based on the sequences of their DNA or RNA and the families of related viruses to which they belong. Clinicians may prefer to classify them by the types of hepatitis they cause, such as a self-limited disease (acute) or a persistent disease (chronic). Epidemiologists may be more interested in the ways they are transmitted. Table 1.1 gives some of the characteristics of the five major human hepatitis viruses.

Table 1.1 The Five Major Human Hepatitis Viruses*

Virus	Genetic Material	Family	Disease	Major Modes of Transmission
Hepatitis A	RNA	Picornaviridae	Acute hepatitis	Contaminated food and water
Hepatitis B	DNA	Hepadnaviridae	Acute and chronic hepatitis	Blood; mother to infant; sex
Hepatitis C	RNA	Flaviviridae	Acute and chronic hepatitis	Blood; mother to infant; sex
Hepatitis D	RNA	Deltaviridae	Acute and chronic hepatitis	Blood (only infects individuals with hepatitis B)
Hepatitis E	RNA	Caliciviridae	Acute hepatitis	Contaminated food and water

*Hepatitis G virus is an RNA virus of the family Flaviviridae that was discovered in 1995. However, it is probably not a major cause of hepatitis.

The distinction between acute and chronic viral hepatitis is important. Some of the human hepatitis viruses, in particular the hepatitis A and E viruses, *only* cause acute disease. Although the acute disease can be quite serious—even fatal—liver inflammation does not persist, and the virus is eliminated from the body as the patient recovers. Some hepatitis viruses, in particular hepatitis B, C, and D (in individuals also infected with the hepatitis B virus), can cause both acute and chronic hepatitis. Chronic hepatitis is defined as hepatitis persisting for more than six months. *Chronicity is the most significant feature of the hepatitis C virus: In the majority of cases, the infection is chronic, usually lasting the patient's lifetime unless it is successfully treated.* Although there are cases in which an individual is infected with the hepatitis C virus and then spontaneously rids the virus from the body and recovers, these cases are relatively rare. In the majority of cases, the patient does not know precisely when he or she was infected, and the hepatitis C virus stays in the body for the patient's lifetime unless treated.

Before the hepatitis C virus was discovered, physicians and scientists had recognized that viral hepatitis was transmitted in two general ways. One type was called *infectious hepatitis* or *epidemic hepatitis*. Outbreaks or epidemics were linked to poor sanitation. The viruses appeared to be spread by eating contaminated food, in particular shellfish, or drinking water contaminated with human feces. The disease was acute, and the infected individuals usually got better; however, about 1 percent of people who contracted hepatitis died. The hepatitis A virus is transmitted in this manner. The hepatitis E virus, which is not present in the United States, is also transmitted in this fashion and causes acute hepatitis in many other parts of the world.

The second type was called *serum hepatitis*. This type was transmitted by blood transfusion or the exchange of blood in other ways, through sexual contact, and from mother to infant. In some cases, in particular with infected infants, it became chronic, with liver inflammation often lasting a patient's lifetime.

In 1965, Dr. Baruch Blumberg and his collaborators discovered a protein in the blood of an Australian aborigine called the Australia antigen. At the time of its discovery, it was not thought to be a viral protein. Over the next few years, however, Dr. Blumberg, his collaborators, and other groups showed that the Australia antigen was associated with serum hepatitis that was transmitted by blood. The Australia antigen was subsequently shown to be the hepatitis B surface antigen (HBsAg). Testing for the presence of HBsAg in the blood is now the most common method for diagnosing hepatitis B virus infection. Blood banks also use this method to screen for infected blood.

By the 1970s, the hepatitis A and B viruses had been identified and fairly well characterized. However, as testing for infection by these two viruses became available, doctors realized that some people with serum hepatitis had no evidence of infection with either the A or B virus. They used the term *non-A, non-B hepatitis* to describe this condition.

Individuals with non-A, non-B hepatitis usually had chronic hepatitis; acute hepatitis was rarely seen after a person received a blood transfusion. Testing of the blood for HBsAg was negative, and patients did not have antibodies against the hepatitis A or B viruses, indicating active infection with them. Most patients with non-A, non-B hepatitis had been exposed to contaminated blood through a blood transfusion or intravenous drug use. There was no evidence for other causes of hepatitis, such as excessive alcohol use, exposure to toxins, metabolic diseases, or autoimmunity.

Evidence from the research laboratory also indicated that a virus caused non-A, non-B hepatitis. If chimpanzees were injected with blood from patients with non-A, non-B hepatitis, they developed hepatitis. Hepatitis could also be transmitted from one chimpanzee to another through blood transfusions. Investigators were so convinced that non-A, non-B hepatitis was caused by an unknown virus that they started clinical trials of interferon alpha, a nonspecific, antiviral agent for treating patients with the condition. Some of the patients with non-A, non-B hepatitis who were treated with interferon alpha showed improvement in their liver inflammation.

This was where hepatology, the study of liver diseases, stood in the late 1980s. At that time, scientists were nearing the discovery of a new virus, which they would later call the hepatitis C virus.

2

Discovery of a New Virus and Its Features

WHEN I WAS a medical student and young physician in training, there was no such thing as hepatitis C. Then in 1989, during my post-doctoral research fellowship at Rockefeller University, a landmark paper was published in the journal *Science*.[1] In this paper, investigators at Chiron Corporation, a relatively new biotechnology company, reported the discovery of a new virus, which they called the hepatitis C virus. In an accompanying paper in the same issue of *Science*,[2] the Chiron scientists and their collaborators showed that about 85 percent of individuals with the diagnosis of non-A, non-B hepatitis had antibodies against portions of the newly discovered virus. In the years since then, millions of individuals have been diagnosed with chronic hepatitis C, and many of them have received treatment. Numerous gastroenterologists and other physicians now consider themselves hepatologists (liver specialists), primarily because of hepatitis C.

The discovery of the hepatitis C virus was based entirely on molecular biology. The Chiron investigators did not isolate a new virus or

---

1. Q-L. Choo et al., "Isolation of a cDNA clone derived from a blood-borne non-A, non-B viral hepatitis genome," *Science* 244 (1989): 359–62.

2. G. Kuo et al., "An assay for circulating antibodies to a major etiological virus of human non-A, non-B hepatitis," *Science* 244 (1989): 362–65.

grow it in the laboratory. In fact, the hepatitis C virus has still not been grown in the laboratory. The Chiron investigators isolated DNA copies of portions of the genetic material of the hepatitis C virus. Based on this discovery, they and others were then able to piece together the entire genome—all the genetic material of the virus. They also produced proteins that comprise the virus and developed the first test for antibodies against the virus in individuals infected with it. The discovery of the hepatitis C virus depended on two assumptions:

1. That the genetic material of a novel virus would be present in chimpanzees infected with blood from human patients with non-A, non-B hepatitis.
2. That blood from patients with non-A, non-B hepatitis would contain antibodies that recognized proteins of this novel virus.

The first step that led to the discovery of the hepatitis C virus was the construction of a DNA "library" of genetic material obtained from chimpanzees infected with blood from a human subject with non-A, non-B hepatitis. Scientists purified or isolated all the DNA and RNA in the blood specimens from the infected chimpanzees because they did not know if the unknown virus had a genome of RNA or DNA. The isolated RNA was copied to DNA using a special enzyme known as reverse transcriptase.[3] The DNA isolated from the monkey's blood and the DNA copies of the purified RNA, known as complementary DNA or cDNA, were then used

---

3. RNA molecules are composed of a chain of sugars (riboses) that are attached to bases with codes U, A, C, G. The sugars attached to these bases are called nucleotides. DNA molecules are composed of a chain of slightly different sugars (deoxyriboses) that are attached to bases with the codes T, A, C, G. Deoxyribose molecules attached to these bases are called deoxynucleotides. The nucleotides and deoxynucleotides in RNA and DNA molecules are linked together in long strands that make up the genetic code. As a result of their chemical properties, a U (in RNA) or a T (in DNA) in one strand can bind to an A in a second strand, and a C can bind to a G. A second RNA or DNA strand in which every G is replaced by a C and every T or U by an A is known as complementary to the first strand. In animals and plants, DNA strands in the genome are copied to complementary RNA strands, which are then translated into amino acids. Some viruses contain RNA molecules as their genome, which depending on the viral species may be copied to complementary RNA or DNA during their life cycles. Since RNA is difficult to work with in certain laboratory experiments, molecular biologists often use a chemical reaction catalyzed by an enzyme known as reverse transcriptase to copy the RNA to a complementary stand of DNA. This DNA can then be used in laboratory experiments in place of the original RNA molecule. The scientist would know that in the complementary DNA, every G would be a C, every C a G, every A a U, and every T an A in the original RNA molecule.

to construct a DNA library. The library contained various pieces of the DNA inserted into a bacteriophage, a special virus that infects bacteria. The infected bacteria were then grown on dishes in the laboratory and treated to induce expression of the various protein pieces encoded by the DNA (see Figure 2.1).

In the second step that led to the discovery of the hepatitis C virus, the blood from patients with non-A, non-B hepatitis was used to isolate bacterial clones infected with bacteriophage that contained proteins encoded by cDNA from the new virus. As discussed previously, blood from infected patients should contain antibodies that recognize proteins of the virus. The new virus was named hepatitis C virus, sometimes abbreviated as HCV. This process is outlined in Figure 2.2.

Figure 2.1 *Construction of a DNA Library from the Blood of Chimpanzees with Non-A, Non-B Hepatitis*

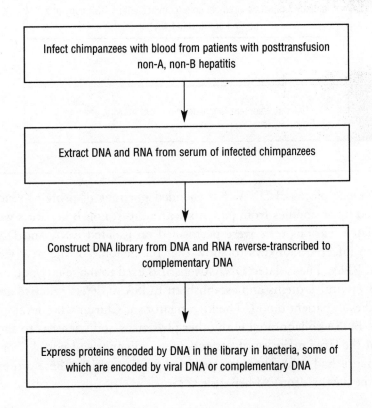

Figure 2.2 Screening of DNA Library with Sera from Patients with Non-A, Non-B Hepatitis

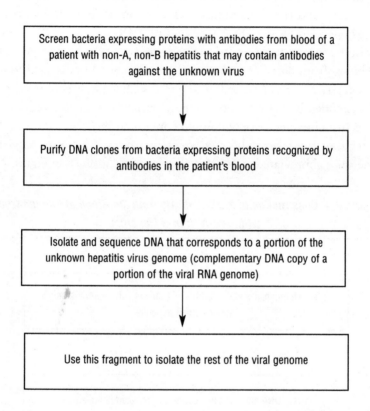

Once pieces of DNA that encoded portions of proteins recognized by antibodies from patients with non-A, non-B hepatitis were isolated, various tests were performed on isolated RNA and DNA from infected monkeys to show that the genome of the new virus was RNA. The isolated DNAs were also used to make large quantities of viral proteins and establish an ELISA to detect reactive antibodies in patient blood. The investigators at Chiron who developed this ELISA collaborated with other physicians and scientists to show that the large majority of patients with a diagnosis of non-A, non-B hepatitis had antibodies in their blood that recognized these proteins of the newly identified hepatitis C virus.

The isolated pieces of DNA corresponding to portions of hepatitis C virus RNA were next used to isolate DNA corresponding to the entire RNA genome. Comparison of the sequence to that of other known viruses showed the new hepatitis C virus to be a member of the Flaviviridae family. Another member of the Flaviviridae family is the yellow fever virus, which also causes liver disease in some parts of the world.

Features of the Hepatitis C Virus

Overall Structure and Composition

The hepatitis C virus genome is composed of 10 kilobases or 10,000 ribonucleotide bases, the building blocks of RNA. This RNA encodes a protein of about 3,030 amino acids, the building blocks of proteins. The large protein encoded by the RNA genome is divided in infected host cells into several smaller structural and nonstructural proteins, schematically illustrated in Figure 2.3.

The functions of the proteins of the hepatitis C virus are briefly described in Table 2.1. Core, E1, and E2 are structural proteins present in the viral particle. Core forms the nucleocapsid (or central core) of the virus with which the RNA genome is associated. The nonstructural (NS) proteins are expressed only in infected cells and

Figure 2.3 A Schematic Diagram Showing the Large Protein Encoded by the Hepatitis C Viral RNA Molecule and Smaller Proteins to Which It Is Processed in Infected Cells

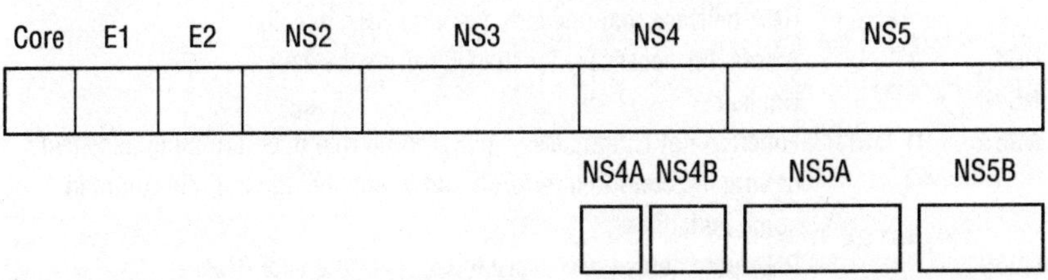

have functions necessary for the replication of the virus. Division of the large protein encoded by the viral RNA is mediated by the action of certain host cell proteins and also the virus's own NS2 and NS3 proteins.

During replication, the hepatitis C virus makes copies of its RNA genome for packaging into viral particles. The NS5B protein is the RNA polymerase that makes copies of the viral RNA. A portion of the NS3 protein unwinds the viral RNA to facilitate replication and protein synthesis. The copied RNA molecules associate with core protein in infected cells and the RNA-associated core protein assembles into viral particles that contain a lipid envelope, derived from intracellular membranes, which contain the E1 and E2 proteins embedded in it.

Although a few reports have been published in which investigators have claimed to see hepatitis C virus particles with an electron microscope, no one has provided conclusive proof. The structure of

Table 2.1 The Proteins of the Hepatitis C Virus

Protein	Function
Structural Proteins	
Core	Forms the viral particle nucleocapsid or core; may have other functions when expressed in host cells such as regulating apoptosis (cell death) and inhibiting cell protein synthesis
E1	Protein of the envelope
E2	Protein of the envelope
P7	Unclear
Nonstructural Proteins	
NS2	A protease that divides the viral polyprotein at a specific site
NS3	A protease that divides the viral polyprotein at specific sites and an RNA-helicase that unwinds the viral RNA in cells
NS4A	A cofactor necessary for the NS3 protease activity
NS4B	Unclear
NS5A	Function not entirely clear; plays some role in determining sensitivity of viral infection to interferon and in enhancing viral replication in some instances
NS5B	RNA-polymerase necessary to replicate the viral RNA

the hepatitis C virus, however, can be inferred from the structures of the proteins encoded by its genetic material and a comparison to other related viruses. The size of the virus is also estimated by passing infected blood through various sized filters before infecting chimpanzees. A schematic diagram of the presumed structure of the hepatitis C virus particle, which circulates in the blood of infected persons, is shown in Figure 2.4.

Genotype

An important feature of each isolate of the hepatitis C virus is its *genotype*. Many liver specialists determine the genotype of the infecting hepatitis C virus as a matter of routine, and patients often have questions about this. What are genotypes? Hepatitis C viruses isolated from different patients show differences in the sequence of their RNA genome. Some of these sequence differences may cause changes in the structures of the encoded proteins. Viral isolates with similar sequences are generally grouped together, and the viral isolates that share certain sequence features belong to a particular genotype. There are six major hepatitis C virus genotypes. These genotypes

Figure 2.4 The Mature Hepatitis C Virus Particle

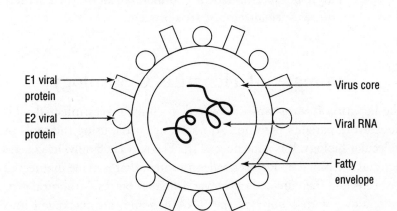

are referred to as genotypes 1 through 6. There are subgenotypes within the major six genotypes, which are referred to by letters: for example, 1a and 1b. Isolates of different genotypes differ enough in their RNA sequence to be classified separately. Those of the same genotype are more similar in their RNA sequence.

Many clinical studies suggest that infection with different hepatitis C virus genotypes may produce different outcomes. Some studies suggest that genotypes 1a and 1b, the most common in the United States, are associated with more aggressive disease and a greater likelihood of progression to cirrhosis, though this conclusion is not certain. Most studies do, however, demonstrate that genotypes 1a and 1b are less likely to respond to treatment with interferon alpha–based therapies.

Quasispecies

Strains of the hepatitis C virus within the same genotype that contain more subtle RNA sequence differences resulting from spontaneous mutations (RNA base changes) are known as *quasispecies*. The virus avoids being eliminated by the immune system by mutating into quasispecies. The emergence of hepatitis C virus quasispecies in an individual with hepatitis C may indicate more aggressive disease and poor response to treatment. At present, quasispecies cannot be determined in commercial laboratories; their detection requires specialized research procedures.

Summary of Hepatitis C Virology

The hepatitis C virus was discovered in chimpanzees infected with blood from patients with non-A, non-B hepatitis, using the tools of molecular biology. It is a member of the Flaviviridae family. Its genetic material is RNA. The RNA encodes a protein that is made in infected host cells and then divided into several smaller pieces. Structural proteins, along with a copy of the RNA genome, are packaged into mature viral particles. These viral particles circulate in the blood of infected individuals and infect liver cells and possibly other cell types.

Nonstructural proteins are expressed only in infected cells and function in various processes, including the replication of the viral RNA and dividing the large protein into smaller fragments. More information on the life cycle of the hepatitis C virus may be found in Chapter 9, which discusses research on potential new drugs.

Based on similarities in the RNA sequence of the genomes of different isolates, the hepatitis C virus is classified into six different genotypes. Type 1 genotypes are the most common in the United States and the most resistant to interferon alpha-based treatments. More subtle RNA sequence differences arising from mutations lead to different quasispecies. Quasispecies development helps the virus evade detection and elimination by the body's immune system.

As of 2001, the hepatitis C virus has not been replicated in cultured cells in the laboratory. Scientists have not been able to infect animals smaller than chimpanzees and humans, which are relatively difficult to study in the research laboratory. Therefore, the development of specific research on drugs to combat hepatitis C has been limited (see Chapter 9). However, isolation and characterization of the genetic material of the hepatitis C virus has allowed scientists to understand something about how the virus infects cells and replicates. It has also made possible the accurate diagnosis of patients with hepatitis C, screening of the blood supply, and a mechanism for following the results of therapy.

3

Transmission of the Hepatitis C Virus

BETWEEN 100 AND 170 million people worldwide are chronically infected with the hepatitis C virus. About 3 to 4 million people are infected in the United States. Hepatitis C virus infection is seen in virtually all parts of the world. In general, the infection rate is higher in more underdeveloped countries. Some countries have an especially high rate, such as Egypt, where more than 10 percent of the population may be infected.

The hepatitis C virus is transmitted primarily via blood, blood products, and tissue or organ transplantation. The two main modes of transmission are by transfusion of contaminated blood or blood products and using unsanitary needles for drug injection. Other less frequent modes of transmission are through sexual contact, from mothers to infants, and through exposure to small quantities of infected blood.

If you casually ask people with hepatitis C to recall instances when they may have been exposed to infection, about a third to a quarter cannot remember one. Even after confidential and focused questioning about past intravenous drug use, about 10 percent of individuals with chronic hepatitis C in the United States still cannot come up with a possible exposure to infection. When discussing risk factors, one must keep in mind that even a single exposure to the virus—even once in the individual's distant past—could have led to infection. A person who shared a needle when using illicit drugs just once in his or her youth or was exposed to a small amount of contaminated blood may be diagnosed with hepatitis C virus infection many years later.

The following are risk factors for developing hepatitis C.

- Transfusion of blood and blood products before 1992 in developed countries[1]
- Organ or tissue transplant before 1992
- Injection of illicit drugs
- Hemodialysis
- Tattooing and body piercing
- Sex with infected partner (higher risk in sexually promiscuous individuals; lower risk in monogamous individuals with infected partner)
- Household (nonsexual) contact with infected individual
- Transmission from infected mother to newborn baby
- Health care and laboratory workers exposed to blood
- Infected health care workers to patients
- Intranasal cocaine use[2]
- Ear piercing in men[2]

Transfusion of Blood and Blood Products

Since 1990, the blood supplies in the United States and most other industrialized countries have been screened for antibodies against the hepatitis C virus. A more sensitive antibody detection test was introduced in 1992, making the risk of getting hepatitis C by transfusion extraordinarily low.

Patients who received blood transfusions before 1990 (and to some extent before 1992), however, are at risk for having hepatitis C.

---

1. Blood supply screening began in developed countries in 1990 and was improved by the introduction of better tests in 1992; those receiving blood transfusions between 1990 and 1992 are still at some risk.

2. It is unclear if these are actually the modes of transmission or factors associated with other lifestyle activities that may increase transmission; for example, intranasal cocaine abusers may also be more likely to have used intravenous drugs at some time.

It has been estimated that since 1992, the chance of receiving a unit of blood contaminated with the hepatitis C virus is less than 1 in 100,000. Hepatitis C is a chronic disease that can last a lifetime; even elderly individuals who received transfusions of blood or blood products long before 1990 can still be infected with the hepatitis C virus. The more units of blood transfused, the higher the risk. The risk is extremely high for individuals who received transfusions of blood products derived from multiple donors. Hemophiliacs who received frequent injections of clotting factors purified from human blood before 1987, when they were treated in a special way to inactivate viruses, have a very high chance of having hepatitis C.

In underdeveloped countries, where the entire blood supply is not screened, the hepatitis C virus may still be transmitted by blood transfusion. This is especially true where individuals may sell their blood, such as poor parts of rural China. In underdeveloped countries, contaminated blood may also be transmitted by the use of unsterile medical equipment in hospitals and doctors' offices. In some parts of the world this is still a likely mode of transmission of the hepatitis C virus.

Organ or Tissue Transplantation

Transplantation of organs from infectious donors to a recipient carried a high risk for transmitting the hepatitis C virus infection before donor screening was available in 1990 and improved in 1992. This includes recipients of heart, kidney, and liver transplants. Currently, this risk is extremely low in developed parts of the world where organ donors are tested for infection with the hepatitis C virus.

Injection of Illicit Drugs

Injection of illicit drugs remains a significant mode of transmission of the hepatitis C virus. Virtually all intravenous drug users share needles and syringes, making direct exposure to other people's blood common. Active intravenous drug users are at an extremely high risk for contracting hepatitis C. Infection rates may be near 90 percent in recurrent urban users.

But even one drug injection in the remote past poses a risk for contracting hepatitis C virus infection. Many individuals are middle-aged when they are first diagnosed with chronic hepatitis C. They may now be upstanding members of the community with important jobs, nice families, and a high standard of living, but used intravenous drugs once or twice "back in the sixties when everyone was using them." For thirty or more years, these patients have lived clean and healthy lives. Little did they know that the hepatitis C virus was lurking in their bodies all during that time.

Other viruses, in particular the hepatitis B virus and HIV, are transmitted by contaminated blood. People who frequently inject illicit drugs have an increased risk of infection with these viruses as well. It is not uncommon for these drug users to have hepatitis B and C, hepatitis C and AIDS, or all three diseases at the same time.

Hemodialysis

Patients with kidney failure may undergo hemodialysis, which is a means of purifying the blood. In hemodialysis, the patient's blood circulates through a machine that removes metabolic waste products and toxins. Although these machines are disinfected after each use, residual blood may be present. Patients with kidney failure are also frequently anemic and may receive blood transfusions while getting hemodialysis. Therefore, hemodialysis, especially before 1990, is a risk factor for hepatitis C. It is also a well-known risk factor for hepatitis B virus infection.

Tattooing and Body Piercing

Tattooing and body piercing are sometimes done with unsterile equipment. Contaminated blood can potentially be transmitted during these procedures. Individuals with tattoos or pierced body parts may therefore be at a slightly increased risk for contracting hepatitis C. This is especially true for people who had these procedures done in underdeveloped countries. One study from the United States has suggested that ear piercing in men, but not in women, is a risk factor for hepatitis C. It's not clear if ear piercing is an actual mode of transmission in the United States, or if men with pierced ears are more likely to have other risk factors for infection than women with pierced ears. Men may also be more likely than women to have their ears pierced in unsterile conditions.

Sexual Transmission

Perhaps the most common questions about the transmission of hepatitis C regard sex. Most studies suggest that individuals with multiple sex partners are at increased risk for infection with the hepatitis C virus. The prevalence of chronic hepatitis C virus infection is significantly higher in promiscuous homosexual men, in patients in sexually transmitted disease clinics, and in female prostitutes than in the general population. This suggests that sexual transmission of the virus is a probable route, although it is not entirely clear if the risk is higher in these groups because of other concurrent lifestyle factors, such as past or current injection drug use. Based on these findings, the Centers for Disease Control and Prevention (CDC) currently recommend that sexually promiscuous individuals should use latex condoms to prevent contracting the hepatitis C virus. This will also prevent transmission of HIV, hepatitis B virus, chlamydia, gonorrhea, syphilis, herpes simplex, and other sexually transmitted pathogens.

Individuals in long-term, monogamous sexual relationships with a partner infected with the hepatitis C virus are at a relatively low risk of becoming infected. Some studies suggest that the sexual partner is at no greater risk for infection than other household contacts. For example, the young son of an infected father has roughly the same risk of getting infected as his mother. Condoms are therefore not considered essential to prevent the spread of the hepatitis C virus for individuals in monogamous sexual relationships with infected partners. Condoms should be considered, however, as the risk of sexual transmission, although very low in monogamous relationships, is still real. Each individual will have to determine his or her own tolerance regarding even this small risk.

Household Contacts of Infected Individuals

Several studies have reported an association between nonsexual household contact and acquiring hepatitis C. This likely occurs as a result of unknown exposure to infectious blood. In the United States, transmission through household contacts is very low. In some other countries, rates as high as 4 percent have been reported.

Transmission from Infected Mother to Newborn Baby

The results of several studies suggest that the rate of transmission of the hepatitis C virus from infected mothers to their newborn babies is about 5 percent. At present, there is no treatment to prevent this. In mothers also infected with the HIV virus, the rate of hepatitis C virus transmission appears significantly higher, at around 15 percent. Women with hepatitis C do not need to avoid pregnancy. However, if a woman has cirrhosis or complications of advanced liver disease, she should discuss the specific risks of pregnancy with her doctor.

Although there is no evidence that the hepatitis C virus is spread by breast-feeding, mothers with hepatitis C should consider not doing this if their nipples are cracked or bleeding. New mothers with hepatitis C should tell their child's pediatrician that they have the disease so that the infant can be appropriately tested for infection and followed accordingly.

Health Care and Public Safety Workers Exposed to Blood

Health care personnel, laboratory workers, emergency medical technicians, and public safety workers exposed to blood in the workplace are at risk for being infected with the hepatitis C virus. However, the prevalence of hepatitis C virus infection among health care workers in the United States appears to be about the same as for the general population. Nonetheless, there are several documented cases of the hepatitis C virus being transmitted to health care workers by their accidentally sticking themselves with infected needles or by other accidents involving exposure to contaminated blood.

Infected Health Care Workers to Patients

The risk for hepatitis C virus transmission from infected health care workers to patients appears to be very low, particularly in the developed world. One report from Spain demonstrated that an infected heart surgeon transmitted the virus to five patients. In this case, transmission occurred during highly invasive open-heart surgery. There have also been rare reports of transmission by contaminated medical equipment; in one case a colonoscope was implicated. These instances are extremely rare, however. No recommendations exist to restrict professional activities of health care workers with hepatitis C virus infection. The usual universal precautions practiced by health care workers when blood and secretions may be exchanged should be followed. In underdeveloped countries where sterile techniques are not routinely practiced, the risk of contracting hepatitis C in the health care setting may be higher.

Intranasal Cocaine

One study has demonstrated that intranasal cocaine use is a risk factor for infection with the hepatitis C virus. Some investigators have hypothesized that the sharing of straws can transmit the virus, as a small amount of bleeding can occur inside the nose while snorting cocaine. This mode of transmission has not been clearly proven, however. It is possible that intranasal cocaine use may only be a surrogate risk factor for hepatitis C virus infection because such individuals are more likely to use, or to have used, intravenous drugs. Nonetheless, intranasal cocaine use should be considered as a possible mode of transmission of the hepatitis C virus.

Prevention and Recommendations Regarding High-Risk Activities

Preventive immunization against the hepatitis C virus is not presently available. However, various prevention activities can reduce or eliminate the risk for hepatitis C virus transmission:

- Screening and testing of blood, organ, tissue, and semen donors
- Viral inactivation of blood-derived products such as clotting factors
- Counseling for people at risk, for example, those using illegal drugs
- Implementation of appropriate infection control practices (such as gloves and gowns) in the health care setting
- Identification and possible treatment of infected individuals
- Public and professional education about hepatitis C virus transmission
- Use of latex condoms by those engaging in high-risk sexual practices

The following are some specific recommendations of the CDC regarding the prevention of hepatitis C:

1. Individuals infected with the hepatitis C virus should be advised not to donate blood, organs, tissue, or semen.
2. Infected persons should not share toothbrushes, dental appliances, razors, or other personal care articles that might have blood on them and should cover cuts and sores to keep from spreading infectious blood or secretions.
3. Persons who use or inject illegal drugs should be advised to stop using and injecting drugs and to enter and complete a substance abuse treatment program.
4. If intravenous drug users continue to inject drugs, they should be counseled to never reuse or share syringes, needles, water, or other drug preparation equipment; if

possible, they should obtain sterile equipment (some cities have syringe and needle exchange programs).

5. Sexually promiscuous persons should be instructed about their risks for hepatitis C and other diseases and be told to use latex condoms correctly every time they have sex to protect themselves and their partners from diseases spread through sexual activity.

6. Health care, emergency medical, public safety, and certain laboratory workers should be educated regarding risk for and prevention of blood-borne infections. They should use standard barrier precautions (such as wearing gloves and gowns). Engineering controls should be implemented to prevent exposure to blood; if health care is provided in the home, the patient's household contacts should be educated about risks of disease transmission and precautions.

7. In chronic hemodialysis settings, intensive efforts must be made to educate new and existing staff regarding hemodialysis-specific, infection-control practices that prevent transmission of the hepatitis C virus and other blood-borne pathogens.

8. Persons considering tattooing or body piercing should be informed of the potential risk of acquiring infection with the hepatitis C virus. Equipment should be sterile, and the artist or piercer should follow other proper infection-control procedures (washing hands, using latex gloves, and cleaning and disinfecting surfaces).

Misconceptions and Recommendations Regarding Low-Risk Activities

Many people have misconceptions about how the hepatitis C virus is spread. First and foremost, it is *not* spread by casual contact. This includes coughing, sneezing, hugging, and kissing; sharing food, eating utensils, or drinking glasses; and contact with toilet seats. It is also *not* spread by mosquitoes. Although household contacts of individuals with hepatitis C are at a modestly increased risk of contracting the virus, this results from exposure to infected blood through sharing razors or toothbrushes and *not* through casual contact. Individuals with hepatitis C should never be excluded from work, school, play, child care, or other similar normal activities. *People with hepatitis C should engage in all usual social and household activities.* However, they should follow the applicable recommendations in this chapter regarding blood exposure and sexual practices.

4

Diagnosis of Hepatitis C

The Silent Disease:
Who Should See a Doctor?

Hepatitis C is sometimes inappropriately called the "silent killer."
This is not an accurate term because it does not kill most of its vic-
tims. However, in most cases hepatitis C is a silent disease. Most
people who are infected with the hepatitis C virus do not know it.
The majority of infected individuals have no symptoms. Most people
with symptoms from chronic hepatitis C have complaints similar to
people with other diseases or, for that matter, healthy people, such
as fatigue, loss of appetite, depression, and joint aches and pains.

Many patients with hepatitis C are diagnosed when they see a
doctor for other reasons. The infection is often first suspected when
an individual undergoes blood testing while applying for health or
life insurance and an abnormal liver test result turns up. Such individuals usually then go to doctors for a diagnosis. In others, hepatitis C virus infection is picked up when they donate blood. Because
hepatitis C is usually asymptomatic, many people who do not routinely see a doctor, get blood tests for other reasons, or donate
blood will not know they are infected with the hepatitis C virus.
For these reasons, some people who may be at risk for hepatitis C

(see Chapter 3) should see a doctor for screening. The at-risk groups of individuals who should be tested for hepatitis C virus infection, according to the Centers for Disease Control and Prevention (CDC), are listed in Table 4.1.

Testing for hepatitis C should be followed by appropriate counseling and medical follow-up. Those who desire testing for hepatitis C virus infection should see a doctor or other primary health care professional. Testing for hepatitis C virus infection outside the primary health care setting should be obtained from a community-based or legitimate health organization that can offer counseling and referral to medical follow-up.

Testing for hepatitis C virus infection is not recommended for all individuals. Less than 1 percent of the overall population in the United States is chronically infected, and routine screening of the

Table 4.1 Individuals Recommended for Testing for the Hepatitis C Virus

- Individuals who have ever injected illegal drugs, including those who injected once many years ago

- Individuals, such as hemophiliacs, who received clotting factor concentrates produced before they were treated for possible viral contamination in 1987

- Individuals who were on long-term hemodialysis

- Individuals with persistent abnormal blood tests suggesting liver disease

- Individuals who received a blood transfusion before July 1992

- Individuals who received an organ transplant before July 1992

- Recipients of blood transfusions or organ transplants who were notified that they received blood from a donor who later tested positive

- Health care, emergency medical, laboratory, and public safety workers after needle sticks, cuts, or mucosal exposures to hepatitis C virus–contaminated blood

- Children born to women infected with the hepatitis C virus

general population should not be performed. It is not clear if this recommendation applies to individuals in all parts of the world where the prevalence of hepatitis C virus infection is much higher. Routine testing for hepatitis C virus infection is not indicated for all health care, emergency medical, and public safety workers unless they know they have been exposed to contaminated blood through accidentally sticking themselves with a needle or cuts from other equipment, or mucosal contact. It is also not indicated for pregnant women or individuals who have household (nonsexual) contact with infected individuals.

There are some groups of individuals for whom routine testing for hepatitis C virus infection may be indicated, but the usefulness of this is currently not clear. People who fall into these groups should probably determine for themselves whether or not to see a doctor for testing. These groups include recipients of transplanted tissues, such as cornea, skin, ova, or sperm. Intranasal cocaine users or drug users who have injected drugs may be at increased risk of having hepatitis C. Persons with numerous tattoos or body piercings, especially those who obtained these in underdeveloped parts of the world, may be at increased risk. Individuals who have had multiple sex partners or a history of a sexually transmitted disease and long-term sex partners of a person with hepatitis C may also be at increased risk for infection (see Chapter 3).

The individual who has an abnormal blood test result indicating a liver problem deserves special mention. This is probably the most common way in which individuals with chronic hepatitis C first become aware of the infection. Many insurance companies do routine blood testing for high levels of serum aminotransferases, which indicate liver disease. Insurance is usually denied to individuals with abnormal results. A high level of serum aminotransferases can indicate a wide range of liver diseases, including alcoholic liver disease and fatty liver, which are more common in the United States than chronic hepatitis C. Elevations in the serum aminotransferase activities are often the first suggestion that a person has chronic hepatitis C. Regardless of the cause of the blood test abnormality, individuals denied insurance because of an abnormal liver blood test should see a doctor for a diagnosis. If the blood test abnormality persists, that individual should be tested for infection with the hepatitis C virus unless another diagnosis is readily apparent to the doctor.

What to Expect When You Visit the Doctor

Infection with the hepatitis C virus can be diagnosed by blood testing alone. However, the accurate and complete diagnosis of any liver disease, including hepatitis C, depends on a combination of obtaining the patient's medical history, examining the patient, and performing laboratory tests and a liver biopsy. Sometimes radiological scans are also necessary. It is hazardous to diagnose a liver disease, especially the extent of the disease and how it may affect the patient, without knowing all this information.

Individuals often call or send me E-mail messages saying that they are infected with the hepatitis C virus, and then include one or two blood test results and ask, "What's my prognosis?" My answer is always: *Only a doctor who obtains a complete history, examines the patient, reviews all the laboratory test results, knows the results of relevant radiological tests, and, in most cases, examines the liver biopsy can answer your question.* There are no exceptions. You must see a doctor for advice regarding your particular case.

Medical History

The cornerstone of medical diagnosis is the patient's history. Without obtaining a complete history, it is difficult for any doctor to make a reliable diagnosis. The history first involves a discussion between the doctor and patient, or a family member, such as a baby's parent or another surrogate, if the patient cannot provide the information. The medical history comprises several parts: the present illness (events and complaints related to why the patient is now seeing the doctor), past medical history, family history, social history, current medications, and allergies. A complete history also includes a review of systems in which the doctor asks the patient about symptoms related to all the different organ systems of the body. In most cases, these separate parts of the history are highly interrelated. For example, a social history of past drug use will also be part of the history of the present illness in someone with chronic hepatitis C.

In addition to asking direct questions, a doctor may obtain part of the history by reviewing the patient's old medical records and test results. A doctor would be particularly interested in seeing the results of past laboratory tests and in reviewing previous radiological scans and liver biopsy slides. Hepatitis C is a chronic disease that is often not diagnosed. Prior to 1990, there was no diagnostic test. Evidence of liver inflammation in previous blood tests would suggest that the patient had hepatitis C as far or further back than the time of the old test result. On their initial visit, patients should bring all available past medical records.

Several aspects of a patient's medical history are of particular importance in diagnosing chronic hepatitis C. Patients should be willing to openly discuss the following issues with their doctors.

- Injection drug use, even if only once long ago
- Use of noninjection drugs
- Tattoos or body piercing
- Sexual activities
- Blood transfusions
- Receipt of blood products such as clotting factors
- Occupational history, especially work in a health care setting
- Travel to or emigration from underdeveloped areas of the world
- Alcohol consumption
- Use of prescription and over-the-counter drugs
- Liver disease in family members
- Past episodes of jaundice (yellow eyes and skin)
- Past blood test results

A complete history from a patient with hepatitis C should include a discussion of common risk factors (see Chapter 3). A frank discussion of past and current drug use is very important. Don't be afraid or embarrassed! Most doctors have heard and seen it all, and none will call the police if you admit to using illegal drugs. Even if you injected an illicit drug only once many years ago, you could be infected with the hepatitis C virus. Openly discuss *any* past drug use with your doctor, including intranasal cocaine use.

Don't be embarrassed to discuss sex with your doctor. The hepatitis C virus can be transmitted by sex, especially in promiscuous individuals (see Chapter 3). A careful sexual history is important to establish how you may have been infected with the hepatitis C virus or other pathogens and if you may be putting others at risk for infection.

An occupational history can establish possible exposure to hepatitis viruses at the workplace. A history of living in certain parts of the world should be ascertained, as hepatitis C and hepatitis B are endemic in some places. Tell your doctor about all your travels, even trips you took many years ago.

Both prescription and over-the-counter drugs can cause liver disease. It is essential for a doctor to obtain a complete drug history from individuals with liver disease and for patients to discuss all the drugs they use. Even if drugs are not the cause of liver disease, drugs may be metabolized differently in patients with advanced liver disease and may contribute to an underlying problem.

Drug and alcohol use must be carefully evaluated in patients with liver diseases, including those with chronic hepatitis C. Alcohol abuse is the leading cause of liver disease in the United States and many other countries. It is generally accepted that individuals infected with hepatitis C who drink significant quantities of alcohol are at an increased risk of developing serious liver disease, such as cirrhosis. Patients should not hide information or lie about the amount of alcohol they drink (though virtually all individuals significantly underreport alcohol consumption). The quantity of alcohol that individuals must consume to acquire liver disease varies tremendously, and the reasons for differences in individual susceptibilities are unknown. However, alcohol should always be considered as a *possible* contributing factor to liver disease, including the severity of chronic hepatitis C, especially in individuals who regularly have more than two drinks a day.

Evaluation of the patient with liver disease, including hepatitis C, also involves a detailed family history. There is approximately a 5 percent chance that an infected pregnant woman may transmit the hepatitis C virus to her newborn baby. The hepatitis B virus is also transmitted from mother to child. Several liver diseases, such as Wilson disease, hemochromatosis, and alpha-1-antitrypsin deficiency, are inherited.

Most patients with chronic hepatitis C have no symptoms or have nonspecific symptoms, such as fatigue, loss of appetite, and depression. Some individuals may have symptoms related to cirrhosis or advanced liver disease when they are first diagnosed. The doctor should ask about symptoms related to advanced liver disease. These include jaundice (yellow skin or eyes), edema (retention of fluid and swelling, usually in the lower extremities), ascites (retention of fluid and swelling in the abdomen), easy bruising or bleeding, confusion, and history of bleeding from the stomach or esophagus. Pruritus, or itching, could also be a symptom of liver disease.

Hepatitis C is one of many liver diseases. A patient may have a different liver disease that is misdiagnosed as hepatitis C. Or a patient may have hepatitis C and another liver disease at the same time. Questions related to other diseases, such as those caused by alcohol, drugs, obesity, or which are inherited, are necessary.

Physical Examination

All patients with chronic hepatitis C should undergo a complete physical examination. The physical examination will sometimes provide clues to the severity of a patient's disease. It will also provide information about the patient's overall physical health, which may be important in making a prognosis and decisions regarding treatment (for example, patients with significant heart disease cannot take ribavirin, a drug used to treat hepatitis C).

Many patients with chronic hepatitis C will have a normal physical examination. Patients generally will not have signs of liver disease unless the liver damage is particularly severe or complications of cirrhosis are present. However, there are several signs of less advanced chronic liver disease that can be detected on physical examination.

A physical examination begins with inspection. In some cases, signs of liver disease may be obvious just by looking at the patient.

Jaundice is yellowing of the eyes, skin, and mucus membranes caused by retention of bilirubin. Bilirubin is normally secreted by the liver into the bile and eliminated from the body. If the liver fails, bilirubin is elevated in the blood, and if its concentration gets above a certain level, it deposits in the eyes, skin, and mucus membranes and gives the patient a yellowish or, when severe, greenish color. Jaundice is usually first detected in the whites of the eyes or under the fingernails, especially in individuals with dark skin. At higher blood concentrations, the inside of the mouth may appear slightly yellowish. In lighter skinned people, jaundice is usually detectable by looking at the skin. Jaundice does not generally occur in chronic hepatitis C unless liver disease is advanced and the person has developed cirrhosis. Jaundice may be a characteristic of other acute or chronic liver diseases and may also be a sign of a disease not involving the liver, such as one causing rapid destruction of red blood cells.

Muscle wasting and weight loss are signs of advanced liver disease and cirrhosis. Every patient with liver disease should be weighed on each visit to the doctor. The muscles should be carefully examined. Excessive and increasing body weight can be a problematic sign in a patient with liver disease. Obesity may cause fatty liver (fat accumulation in the liver cells that can cause inflammation). Fluid retention in cirrhosis can lead to weight gain, and weight should be regularly followed in individuals with cirrhosis. Weight loss may also be observed in patients with significant liver disease.

The doctor should pay careful attention to those parts of the physical examination that may indicate the presence of liver disease. The patient's hands should be examined for Depuytren's contracture, a shortening and thickening under the skin of the palm that can cause the middle fingers to bend. Individuals with cirrhosis or alcohol liver disease may have this. Some patients with liver disease may have "liver palms," or *palmar erythema*, which are palms that are abnormally red in color. Some individuals with chronic or severe liver disease will also have small vascular lesions called "spiders," or more precisely *spider angiomata*. Spider angiomata are small, red dots with "legs" that radiate from the center. They blanch when compressed and turn red again when pressure is released. These are usually found on the arms, shoulders, chest, and back and are virtually never found below the waistline.

Examination of the head and eyes and mouth should be performed. Jaundice may first be apparent in the whites of the eyes and mucus membranes of the mouth. Some individuals with liver disease, especially those with alcoholic cirrhosis, may have enlarged salivary (parotid) glands on the side of the face.

Examination of the abdomen is of central importance. Protrusion of the abdomen may result from fluid retention. Some individuals with cirrhosis will have an umbilical hernia that sticks out of the belly button and can be temporarily pushed in by the doctor. The doctor should feel for the edge of the liver on the upper right side of the abdomen under the ribs, as the liver may be enlarged or abnormal in texture. The doctor should feel for the spleen in the left upper portion of the abdomen. The spleen should not be felt in normal individuals but may be swollen in patients with liver disease. The doctor may also use percussion to estimate the size of the liver. In percussion, the doctor drums on the abdomen and listens for changes in sound from dull to more hollow, air-filled sounds, which occur at the edges of the liver. Liver disease can cause the liver to be either enlarged (*hepatomegaly*) or shrunken. The doctor may feel around the abdomen for the presence of retained fluid, which can be detected by percussion of the flanks. The doctor should also look at the legs and ankles for evidence of fluid retention.

An examination of the nervous system is important in the evaluation of a patient with liver disease. Patients with severe acute liver disease or cirrhosis may have *hepatic encephalopathy*, which causes mental changes ranging from mild confusion to deep coma. The first change in mental capacity is the inability to construct simple objects, such as a six-point star using twelve toothpicks. Patients with early hepatic encephalopathy may have difficulty with connect-the-dots drawings. In cases of severe hepatic encephalopathy, marked confusion can occur and patients may have a "liver flap" (*asterexis*). To test for asterexis, the patient is asked to hold up his or her hand like a police officer stopping traffic. If asterexis is present, the hand drops repeatedly or flaps.

Most of the physical signs of liver disease occur in patients with severe acute liver disease and advanced cirrhosis; however, most individuals with chronic hepatitis C will *not* have signs of liver disease. Nevertheless, a careful physical examination is essential for all patients with chronic hepatitis C to check for signs of liver disease and to evaluate the patient's overall state of health.

Laboratory Tests

Blood Testing

Blood testing plays a critical role in the diagnosis of hepatitis C. Tests for antibodies against the virus and for viral RNA in the blood are used to establish that a person is infected. Blood testing is also very important in estimating the extent of liver inflammation and assessing liver function. However, it is only part of the picture and blood test results mean little separate from the history and physical examination. Patients must remember that doctors treat the patient, *not* the test results! Many patients, for example, ask me what they should do to "lower their liver enzymes." My answer is "nothing." You treat the underlying disease.

Blood tests can be broken down into five general categories:

1. Tests to establish infection with the hepatitis C virus
2. Tests to rule out or establish the presence of other liver diseases
3. Tests that detect damage to liver cells and liver inflammation
4. Tests that tell something about liver function
5. Tests that tell something about other organ systems and the patient's overall state of health

Tests to Establish Infection with the Hepatitis C Virus

Two types of tests are used to establish infection with the hepatitis C virus: tests for antibodies against the virus and tests for viral RNA (Table 4.2). The antibody tests are easier to perform, less expensive,

Table 4.2 Blood Tests for Hepatitis C Virus Infection

Antibody Tests

Enzyme-linked immunosorbent assay (ELISA)
Recombinant immunoblot assay (RIBA)

RNA Tests

Reverse transcription–polymerase chain reaction (PCR)
Branched-chain DNA (bDNA)

and generally used for screening and initial diagnosis. The viral RNA tests are more difficult to perform and significantly more expensive. RNA testing is generally used to follow patients who are treated and to establish or rule out infection in patients with confounding histories or other laboratory test results.

Antibody Tests   When a person is infected with a virus, the body's immune system produces antibodies against the virus. The antibody test establishes that a person was exposed to the virus. In the case of hepatitis C, the vast majority of patients with positive antibody tests are actively infected with the virus. Similarly, about 99 percent of patients chronically infected with the hepatitis C virus have a positive antibody test. A positive antibody test in a person with a known risk factor for hepatitis C is essentially diagnostic for chronic hepatitis C, with rare exceptions.

The first test widely available in the diagnosis of hepatitis C virus infection was the enzyme-linked immunosorbent assay, or ELISA. The ELISA is used for detecting antibodies against proteins of the hepatitis C virus. Since it first became available in 1990, the ELISA has been repeatedly improved. A significiantly improved ELISA introduced in 1992 made the diagnosis of chronic hepatitis C reliable and the blood supply safe. The currently available ELISAs for hepatitis C are positive in approximately 99 percent of individuals chronically infected with the virus.

In the ELISA, several viral proteins are coated on a plastic dish. The patient's serum (blood containing antibodies but no blood cells) is incubated in the dish. The dish is then rinsed to remove substances that do not bind tightly to the viral proteins. If the patient has anti-bodies against hepatitis C viral proteins, they will stick to the viral proteins coated on the dish. A second antibody, which recognizes human antibodies and has been chemically modified so that it can be readily detected, is then added. This second antibody is used to detect the presence of the first antibody. The ELISA will be positive in virtually all cases of chronic hepatitis C. It will be negative in *acute* hepatitis C, as it takes six weeks or longer for an infected person to develop antibodies.

The ELISA is the first test that most doctors use in the diagnosis of chronic hepatitis C. It is also the test used to screen the blood supply, and donated blood that tests positive in this assay is discarded. *It should be assumed that an individual with a positive ELISA has chronic hepatitis C until proven otherwise.*

In rare cases, the ELISA test for antibodies against the hepatitis C virus can be false positive. False positive means that the test is positive even though the patient does not have hepatitis C. This occurs if antibodies indiscriminately stick to the plastic dish or to any protein. This rare occurrence should be suspected in individuals who have normal liver blood tests and no risk factors. In individuals with a positive hepatitis C ELISA test, a confirmatory RNA test should be performed. A false positive test should also be suspected in individuals with rare diseases that cause elevations in the immunoglobulins in the blood. Autoimmune hepatitis can elevate immunoglobulins and is sometimes confused with hepatitis C. In individuals with a positive hepatitis C ELISA and elevated blood immunoglobulins, a confirmatory RNA test should be performed.

The recombinant immunoblot assay, or RIBA, can determine the exact viral proteins recognized by the antibodies. Since tests for viral RNA have become more widely available, the RIBA is rarely used. In the RIBA, several proteins of the hepatitis C virus are coated onto a plastic strip. A control or irrelevant protein is added to the same strip. The strip is incubated with the patient's blood and processed similarly to the ELISA. If the patient has antibodies that react with two viral proteins and not with the control protein, it is considered positive. If the patient's blood contains antibodies that react with no proteins or the control protein only, it is considered negative. If the patient's blood contains antibodies that react with only one viral protein, or more than one viral protein and the control protein, it is indeterminate. Like the ELISA, the RIBA will also be negative in acute hepatitis C infection.

RNA Tests   Commercial availability of tests to detect hepatitis C virus RNA in blood has changed the way many doctors diagnose hepatitis C virus infection. These tests are for a part of the virus itself. The most sensitive test is reverse transcription–polymerase chain reaction, or RT-PCR, commonly called PCR. In this test, viral RNA is extracted from the blood and copied to DNA by the enzyme, reverse transcriptase. A biochemical reaction known as the polymerase chain reaction (PCR) is then used to amplify the viral DNA copy so that it can be detected by routine chemical methods.

Another test for hepatitis C viral RNA in the blood is the branched-chain DNA assay, commonly called bDNA. In this test, a fraction of the blood is incubated with a synthetic DNA molecule that binds to hepatitis C viral RNA. If viral RNA is present, it is captured in a tiny dish and then detected by a chemical reaction involving a second synthetic DNA molecule. The bDNA test is less often used than PCR, which is more sensitive and can detect lower levels of viral RNA.

Both PCR and bDNA can be used to estimate viral load, the concentration of viral RNA in the blood. Although it is not entirely clear how viral load correlates with prognosis or response to treatment, many doctors and patients focus on this number. I usually tell patients that the most important aspect of the PCR test is whether the viral RNA is or is not detected (positive or negative). I have less to say about the numbers put on the values, although some studies have suggested that a higher viral load may correlate with a lesser chance of responding to treatment. More research is needed.

PCR testing can also be modified or combined with special chemical methods to determine the genotype of the infecting virus. Many liver specialists determine the genotype of the infecting hepatitis C virus as a matter of routine. (The concept of viral genotype is explained in Chapter 2.) There are six major hepatitis C virus genotypes. In the most commonly used nomenclature, they are referred to as genotypes 1 through 6. There are subgenotypes within the major six genotypes, referred to by letters; for example, 1a and 1b. Isolates of different genotypes differ enough in RNA sequence to be grouped separately from each other. In the United States, between 50 and 80 percent of the hepatitis C viral isolates are genotype 1a or 1b. How viral genotype may impact prognosis and treatment is discussed in the next chapter.

RNA tests are *not* screening tests. One role of RNA tests is to confirm or refute the results of an antibody test. In these instances, the PCR is probably a better choice than the bDNA test, as it is more sensitive. If an antibody test is negative and the clinical suspicion of chronic hepatitis C is low—for example, in a person with no apparent risk factors and normal blood test results—the patient very likely does not have chronic hepatitis C. However, if the doctor strongly suspects hepatitis C despite a negative antibody test, a PCR test should be performed because patients infected with the hepatitis C virus occasionally have negative antibody tests. PCR testing is also a good idea to confirm or rule out chronic hepatitis C in patients for whom an antibody test may be falsely positive, such as those with high concentrations of blood immunoglobulins. An RNA test should probably be performed in a patient with a positive antibody test but no risk factor for hepatitis C virus infection and normal blood test results. An RNA test must also be performed in suspected cases of acute hepatitis C, as antibody tests will be negative in those cases.

Hepatitis C virus RNA tests are mainly used for checking responses to treatment. PCR, or possibly bDNA, should probably be performed prior to treatment. Some doctors will perform follow-up tests after two to six months of treatment to determine if the patient has responded. A patient is considered to have responded if viral RNA is no longer detectable in blood. Whether or not such testing should be performed during treatment and at what particular intervals has not been conclusively established. However, RNA testing, preferably the more sensitive PCR, should definitely be performed six months after stopping treatment and perhaps periodically thereafter. Negative tests for hepatitis C viral RNA six months or longer after treatment is now generally considered the definition of a sustained response.

Tests to Rule Out or Establish the Presence of Other Liver Diseases

Hepatitis C virus infection can cause hepatitis, which is inflammation of the liver. Other viruses, drugs, alcohol, autoimmune disorders, inherited diseases of metabolism, circulatory problems, toxins, and excessive fat in liver cells can also cause hepatitis. The patient with hepatitis C may also have one of these other conditions, or a patient presumed to have hepatitis C may actually have one of these conditions and not hepatitis C. Most patients who are eventually diagnosed with chronic hepatitis C first come to medical attention because of abnormalities in blood tests that detect liver cell damage and inflammation, but not the causes. Therefore, a doctor who first sees a patient with hepatitis usually considers other diagnoses in addition to hepatitis C.

Just as a careful medical history and physical examination can strongly suggest a diagnosis of hepatitis C or make it seem unlikely, they can also exclude many of the other common causes of hepatitis. Sometimes special blood testing is needed to exclude or establish these diagnoses. Table 4.3 outlines some of the blood tests that a doctor may order, depending on the patient's history, to help diagnose various types of liver diseases.

In obvious cases of hepatitis C, most of these blood tests will not be necessary to determine alternative or concurrent causes of liver inflammation. However, the hepatitis B virus, which can also chronically infect the liver, is transmitted in similar fashion to the hepatitis C virus. Therefore, patients with chronic hepatitis C and past exposure to blood, such as injection drug users, should also be tested for infection with the hepatitis B virus. Appropriate blood tests for the hepatitis A and B viruses could also establish *past* infections with these viruses to which the individual is now immune. This will provide useful information regarding possible vaccination for hepatitis A and B.

Table 4.3 Laboratory Tests for Viral, Autoimmune, and Metabolic Liver Diseases

Condition	Test
Viral Hepatitis	
Hepatitis A	Antibodies against viral proteins for past or current infection
Hepatitis B	Antibodies against viral proteins for evidence of past or current infection; test for viral protein or DNA in blood for current infection
Hepatitis C	Antibodies against viral proteins and presence of viral RNA in blood for current infection
Hepatitis D	Antibodies against viral proteins for current infection
Hepatitis E	Antibodies against viral proteins for past or current infection
Autoimmune Diseases	
Autoimmune hepatitis	"Autoantibodies" against proteins from cell nuclei (antinuclear antibodies) and smooth muscle cells (antismooth muscle antibodies); serum protein electrophoresis for elevated gamma-globulin
Metabolic Diseases	
Hemochromatosis	Iron, transferrin, and ferritin concentrations in blood
Wilson disease	Ceruloplasmin concentration in blood and urine copper concentrations
Alpha-1-antitrypsin deficiency	Alpha-1-antitrypsin concentration in blood

Tests That Detect Damage to Liver Cells and Liver Inflammation

Aminotransferases, also sometimes referred to as *transaminases*, are enzymes that facilitate certain chemical reactions within cells. Two major aminotransferases are present in hepatocytes, the primary liver cells. These are alanine aminotransferase (ALT) and aspartate aminotransferase (AST). The older names for these enzymes, still used by some doctors and clinical laboratories, were SGPT and

SGOT, respectively. ALT is present primarily in hepatocytes, and AST is present in hepatocytes as well as in the cells of some other tissues, such as heart and skeletal muscle.

ALT and AST leak out from dead or damaged cells and into the bloodstream. As a result, their activities in the blood can be measured. Activity is a unit of measurement used by biochemists that is roughly proportional to amount. In healthy individuals, the activities (amounts) of ALT and AST in the blood fall into normal ranges that vary slightly from one laboratory to another. When hepatocyte damage or death is increased, such as in liver inflammation (hepatitis), ALT and AST leak out of the cells at greater rates and their activities are increased in the blood. ALT and AST are indications of inflammation and increased hepatocyte damage and possible death.

Many doctors, nurses, and patients refer to ALT and AST as liver function tests. This is unfortunate because blood ALT and AST activities do *not* relate to the liver's *function*. Some people refer to them as liver enzymes, a more accurate but still imprecise term, as there are many other enzymes in liver cells, some of which are also measured in the clinical laboratory. I have tried for many years to stop doctors and medical students from using the term *liver function tests* for blood ALT and AST. The activities of ALT and AST in blood are abnormally elevated when liver cells are damaged or dead, often as a result of ongoing inflammation. However, the blood ALT and AST activities can be absolutely normal in a liver that is hardly functioning. Similarly, they can be significantly elevated when there is liver inflammation or cell death despite the fact that liver function is preserved.

Elevations in blood ALT and AST activities are often the first indicator that someone has chronic hepatitis C or any other type of hepatitis. Measurement of ALT and AST is often included in many routine blood test panels ordered by doctors. They are also checked as part of many life or health insurance examinations. As people with chronic hepatitis frequently do not have any symptoms, elevations in one or both of these blood tests is very often how a person first finds out that he or she may have hepatitis. Evaluation of blood ALT and AST is usually why most patients with hepatitis C first see a doctor.

Blood ALT and AST activities are both elevated to approximately equal levels in chronic hepatitis, including hepatitis C. Sometimes one will be more elevated than the other; sometimes one is normal while the other is slightly elevated. Any of these situations should suggest the presence of liver inflammation. One interesting situation is alcoholic hepatitis where, for unclear reasons, the blood AST activity is often more highly elevated than the ALT activity. Blood AST activity, and sometimes ALT activity, can also be elevated in nonliver conditions, such as heart attack and skeletal muscle damage, as these enzymes, particularly AST, are also present in the cells of these tissues.

Blood aminotransferase activities are elevated in many different liver diseases. In chronic hepatitis from any cause, they are usually less than ten times normal, but in some cases may be higher. ALT and AST are also elevated in cases of acute liver cell death caused by shock, drugs, toxins, viral hepatitis, or other insults.

The degree of elevation of blood AST and ALT activities roughly, but not exactly, approximates the amount of liver cell death from inflammation or other causes. However, some individuals with hepatitis can have significant inflammation and only mild elevations of blood aminotransferase activities. Rarely, some individuals can have very high blood ALT and AST activities and only mild inflammation in their liver biopsies. This is particularly true for chronic hepatitis C.

Following are important things to remember about blood AST and ALT, particularly in regard to hepatitis C:

- They are often the first blood test abnormalities that indicate that a person may have chronic hepatitis C.
- They are not specific for hepatitis C and can be elevated in many different liver diseases where liver cell death from inflammation or other causes occurs. Elevations in blood ALT and AST activities are *not* specific for any particular diagnosis and further evaluation is necessary.
- AST and ALT activities are absolutely *not* liver function tests. Blood ALT and AST activities may be high in someone with preserved liver function. On the other hand, they can be normal in someone with end-stage cirrhosis and virtually no remaining liver function.

- Elevations of blood ALT and AST activities strongly suggest the presence of liver disease and should be evaluated by a doctor. In some cases, the liver disease will turn out to be hepatitis C.
- People found to be infected with the hepatitis C virus by screening should have their blood ALT and AST activities measured to assess possible liver inflammation.
- In individuals with a chronic liver disease, including hepatitis C, blood ALT and AST are *approximate* markers of the degree of liver inflammation or liver cell death. However, it must be stressed again that some individuals with normal ALT and AST activities may have significantly advanced liver disease and even cirrhosis while some with elevated values may have minimal inflammation.

Two other enzymes must be mentioned when discussing blood tests related to liver cell damage. These are alkaline phosphatase and gamma-glutamyltranspeptidase (GGTP). Alkaline phosphatase is found in many different cells of the body, including those lining the large and small bile ducts within the liver. Alkaline phosphatase is also prominently present in cells of the kidney, intestine, bone, and placenta in pregnant women. Blood alkaline phosphatase activity can be elevated in disorders involving any of these tissues. GGTP, on the other hand, is present almost exclusively in the parts of the hepatocytes that secrete bile and the bile duct cells.

Elevations in blood alkaline phosphatase and GGTP activities, especially when ALT and AST activities are normal or only modestly elevated, suggest bile duct disease or abnormal bile flow. These can be diseases of either the large bile ducts outside the liver—for example, obstruction by a gallstone or cancer—or of the tiny bile ducts within the liver. Many drugs also cause stagnation of bile flow and resultant elevations in the blood alkaline phosphatase and GGTP activities. In liver diseases not directly affecting the bile ducts, such as hepatitis C, the blood alkaline phosphatase and GGTP activities may also be elevated. In these diseases, however, elevations are usually modest, and ALT and AST activities are elevated to a more significant degree. In contrast, liver diseases that primarily affect the bile ducts are characterized by more marked elevations in the blood alkaline phosphatase and GGTP activities, and only modestly elevated or normal blood ALT and AST activities. Blood GGTP activity may also be elevated in individuals without structural liver disease who drink too much alcohol or take certain drugs or medications. Blood GGTP can sometimes be elevated in individuals without liver disease who do not drink alcohol or take medications.

As is the case with aminotransferase activities, elevations in the blood alkaline phosphatase or GGTP activities are *not* diagnostic for any specific disease. Their elevations suggest disorders of the bile ducts or bile flow. They may also be elevated to a lesser degree than ALT and AST in liver diseases that primarily affect hepatocytes, such as hepatitis C. In very unusual cases of hepatitis C, the blood alkaline phosphatase and/or GGTP may be elevated, while the ALT and AST are normal or very near normal. More commonly, their elevations suggest disorders of the bile ducts.

The blood lactate dehydrogenase (LDH) may also be elevated in patients with liver disease. LDH is a nonspecific test that can be elevated in many different conditions, including blood diseases and lung diseases. Although LDH may be elevated in liver disease, testing LDH levels is rarely used to determine liver cell damage because of its low specificity compared to the aminotransferases.

Tests That Tell Something About Liver Function

Liver enzyme tests such as ALT, AST, GGTP, and alkaline phosphatase are *not* liver function tests. However, there are some laboratory tests that do tell something about liver function. Three of the most important ones are blood bilirubin concentration, blood albumin concentration, and prothrombin time. The complete blood count and the ammonia concentration may also tell something about the status of the liver's function. None of these tests, however, are specific for liver function, and they can be abnormal in diseases and conditions that affect other organs. Abnormalities in these tests in patients with liver diseases do suggest that the liver function may be abnormal.

In chronic hepatitis C, the liver generally continues to function normally until the patient develops cirrhosis. Therefore, blood tests that tell something about liver function are usually normal in someone with chronic hepatitis C unless the disease is advanced. In chronic hepatitis C, cirrhosis generally does not develop until many years after infection, and in fact, most individuals with chronic hepatitis C will never develop cirrhosis. Therefore, most people with chronic hepatitis C will have normal blood tests that tell something about liver function. Those with abnormalities suggest that cirrhosis has developed. However, they can all be normal for patients with early-stage cirrhosis.

The following list gives some of the major functions of the liver. This list gives some idea as to why blood tests such as the bilirubin concentration, albumin concentration, and prothrombin time (a test of blood clotting) can be abnormal as the liver begins to function abnormally. (For more information on normal liver function, I refer readers to *The Liver Disorders Sourcebook*.)

- Conjugation and secretion of bilirubin
- Synthesis and secretion of albumin
- Synthesis of blood-clotting factors
- Cholesterol and fatty acid metabolism
- Glucose (simple sugar) and carbohydrate (complex sugar) metabolism
- Detoxification of various harmful substances
- Metabolism of many drugs and alcohol
- Synthesis of bile salts
- Protein metabolism

Bilirubin   Bilirubin comes primarily from the breakdown of old red blood cells. A small fraction also comes from the breakdown of proteins in other organs. The normal red blood cell life is about one hundred twenty days in the body. Specialized cells, primarily in the spleen, take up the dying red blood cells and destroy them. Hemoglobin, the major red blood cell protein that carries oxygen in the blood, is then chemically converted to bilirubin, which is greenish-yellow in color.

Bilirubin is extremely insoluble in water and circulates in the bloodstream bound to the protein albumin. Bilirubin-bound albumin taken up from the blood by the liver. In the hepatocytes, bilirubin is chemically converted by a process called *conjugation* into a more water-soluble form. In conjugation, bilirubin undergoes a chemical reaction with a water-soluble compound called *glucuronic acid*. As a result of this chemical reaction, two glucuronic acid molecules are usually attached to one bilirubin molecule to create a compound known as *bilirubin diglucuronide*. Bilirubin diglucuronide is generally referred to as *conjugated bilirubin*.

Conjugated bilirubin is secreted from the hepatocytes into the very tiny bile ducts within the liver. These tiny bile ducts merge into larger bile ducts that eventually form the common bile duct that empties into the small intestine. In a healthy liver, almost all the conjugated bilirubin is secreted into the bile and only a very small amount leaks out of hepatocytes back into the bloodstream. As a result of conjugation in the liver and secretion into the bile, the total blood bilirubin concentration in normal individuals is usually less than 17 micromolar, or about 1 milligram per deciliter.

If the liver functions improperly, there is a deficiency of bilirubin secretion into the bile and its concentration increases in the blood. When bilirubin in the blood is measured in the clinical laboratory, values for direct and total bilirubin are usually reported. The direct bilirubin roughly represents the more water-soluble conjugated bilirubin. The total bilirubin in the blood is the sum of the conjugated and unconjugated bilirubin. Most of the total bilirubin in the blood is the unconjugated bilirubin that is produced from hemoglobin and other proteins prior to being conjugated in the liver. The estimate of the unconjugated bilirubin, usually calculated as the total bilirubin minus direct bilirubin, is called the indirect bilirubin.

In acquired liver diseases such as cirrhosis from hepatitis C, the secretion of conjugated bilirubin from the liver cells into the bile is affected. Such patients will have elevations primarily in the direct bilirubin, with the total bilirubin also elevated. As an acquired liver disease progresses, both the direct and indirect bilirubin concentrations can be elevated.

The conversion of bilirubin to its more water-soluble form by conjugation in the liver enables it to be more readily filtered by the kidneys and secreted in the urine. If the concentration of conjugated bilirubin in the blood becomes too high, it can be detected in the urine. In such instances, the urine may appear dark yellow or brown in color.

An elevated concentration of bilirubin in the blood is known as *hyperbilirubinemia*. The normal bilirubin concentration in the blood is less than 17 micromolar, or about 1 milligram per deciliter. When the blood bilirubin exceeds 35 micromolar, or about 2 milligrams per deciliter, jaundice becomes apparent. As the blood bilirubin concentration gets higher, a patient may appear very yellow in color.

Elevations in blood bilirubin are *not* specific for cirrhosis from advanced hepatitis C. Blood bilirubin concentrations can be elevated in cirrhosis of any cause and in acute liver diseases that subsequently resolve. The direct bilirubin can be elevated in bile duct obstruction. A gallstone blocking the bile duct is one of the most common causes of jaundice in adults.

Indirect bilirubin is elevated in the blood in a fairly common condition known as Gilbert syndrome. In Gilbert syndrome, either the uptake of unconjugated bilirubin from the blood or its conjugation in liver cells is slightly impaired. Patients with Gilbert syndrome may become jaundiced under times of stress or fasting. Gilbert syndrome is common, and patients with chronic hepatitis C may also have it. Gilbert syndrome is *not* a disease and does not require treatment. The diagnosis is made if the indirect (unconjugated) bilirubin is elevated, and there is no cause of excessive production such as increased red blood cell breakdown.

Indirect bilirubin concentrations in the blood can also be elevated in diseases that do not affect the liver. The blood indirect bilirubin may be elevated in conditions that cause red blood cells to be rapidly destroyed in the body. Even an injury producing a very large hematoma, or bruise, can cause the bilirubin to be temporarily elevated.

Important things to remember about blood bilirubin concentration in regard to hepatitis C are:

- It is usually normal until cirrhosis is present.
- The direct (conjugated) bilirubin is usually primarily elevated in cirrhosis from hepatitis C.
- Elevations in blood bilirubin are not specific for cirrhosis from hepatitis C, or even for liver disease.
- Blood bilirubin may be elevated in many different liver diseases and also in some nonliver disorders.
- A person with chronic hepatitis C may have elevated blood bilirubin concentrations for other reasons (for example, Gilbert syndrome).

Albumin   Albumin, the most abundant protein in the blood, is synthesized in the liver hepatocytes and secreted into the blood. If liver function is abnormal, the blood albumin concentration may fall. This usually occurs in patients with cirrhosis. The albumin concentration in the blood can also be low in conditions other than liver diseases, including serious malnutrition, kidney diseases, and intestinal disorders. A low albumin concentration in the blood is sometimes referred to as *hypoalbuminemia*. Hypoalbuminemia in a patient with a chronic liver disease suggests that cirrhosis is present and that the liver has begun to function abnormally.

The blood albumin is measured in a test known as the serum protein electrophoresis. In this test the major proteins in the blood are separated in an electric field and their concentrations are measured. The serum proteins measured in this test are albumin, alpha-globulins, beta-globulins, and gamma-globulins. In some cases of cirrhosis, the gamma-globulins may be elevated while the albumin is low. Elevation in the gamma-globulins may also suggest other diseases, such as autoimmune hepatitis.

Prothrombin Time (PT)   Several blood-clotting factors are made in the liver. When liver function is compromised, the synthesis of these blood-clotting factors may be decreased. The prothrombin time (PT) is a blood-clotting test that measures the function of several blood-clotting factors. It is usually reported in seconds or as the international normalized ratio (INR), a ratio of the measured prothrombin time to a standard. The PT is prolonged when the blood concentrations of clotting factors made by the liver are low. In chronic liver diseases, the PT is usually not significantly prolonged until cirrhosis has developed and the amount of liver damage is significant. In acute liver diseases, the PT can be prolonged, with severe, sudden liver damage, and return to normal as the patient recovers. Elevations in the PT can be prolonged in other conditions, such as vitamin K deficiency and inherited or acquired blood-clotting disorders. Drugs such as warfarin (Coumadin), which is used therapeutically as an anticoagulant, also prolong PT.

Complete Blood Count   The complete blood count (CBC) is an important laboratory test in many different patients, including those with liver diseases. Although the CBC is not specific for liver problems, abnormalities may be detected when liver function becomes abnormal. Individuals with chronic liver disease, especially cirrhosis, can be anemic, which would be manifested by low blood hemoglobin concentrations and low hematocrits. The hemoglobin and hematocrit are proportional to the number of red blood cells in a given volume of blood. Patients with cirrhosis can also have decreased numbers of white blood cells, the blood cells that fight infections. Perhaps the most important part of the CBC in individuals with liver disease is the platelet count. Platelets are the smallest of the blood cells and are necessary for normal blood clotting. In individuals with cirrhosis, or in some with very severe, acute liver disease, the spleen can become enlarged as blood flow through the liver is impeded. As a result, platelets may become trapped in the enlarged spleen and the platelet count will fall. In a patient with chronic liver disease, a low platelet count, known as *thrombocytopenia*, suggests that the person might have cirrhosis. However, low platelet counts are *not* specific for liver diseases and can be observed in many different diseases and conditions.

Ammonia   When the liver fails, blood ammonia concentrations may increase. This occurs in severe acute liver disease and in cirrhosis, including cirrhosis that results from chronic hepatitis C. Ammonia is absorbed from the large intestine where it is generated through the breakdown of proteins by bacteria living there. Ammonia is not effectively removed from the blood by the failing liver. As a result, the concentration of ammonia in the blood increases. Blood ammonia concentrations can be elevated in conditions other than liver failure, including some rare metabolic disorders.

Glucose   The blood glucose, or sugar, can be abnormal in liver disease. In severe acute liver failure or very advanced cirrhosis, the blood glucose can be lower than normal. Earlier stage cirrhosis is often associated with diabetes mellitus, causing the blood glucose concentration to be higher than normal. In most patients with chronic hepatitis C and no cirrhosis, the blood glucose is not affected unless they have another condition such as diabetes.

Cholesterol   The blood cholesterol concentration can be low in patients with advanced cirrhosis. It can be elevated in patients with bile duct obstruction or bile duct diseases such as primary biliary cirrhosis. Hepatitis C itself, unless it is the cause of advanced cirrhosis, does not affect the blood cholesterol.

Testing Other Organ Systems and Overall State of Health

Other organ systems besides the liver can be affected as a result of having chronic hepatitis C. The kidneys can be damaged in some cases of hepatitis C because of a condition known as *cryoglobulinemia*. Abnormal kidney function can also occur in patients with cirrhosis. This is detected by elevations in the blood creatinine concentration and the blood urea nitrogen (BUN) concentration. These laboratory results are abnormal in any type of kidney disease. The precise cause of kidney dysfunction in a person with hepatitis C requires additional testing. A urinalysis is usually the first test in helping to establish the possible cause of a kidney disease. The take-home message for patients with hepatitis C is that abnormalities in the blood creatinine or BUN indicate kidney problems that may or may not be caused by hepatitis C. Further evaluation is required to determine the cause.

Tests for cryoglobulinemia deserve discussion in regard to chronic hepatitis C. This condition is defined by the presence of cryoglobulins in the blood. *Cryoglobulin* is a term for proteins in the blood that precipitate out at cold temperatures. The test for cryoglobulins involves placing a tube of blood in a refrigerator (actually serum, which is blood minus the blood cells) and seeing if proteins that are soluble at room temperature come out of the solution. In chronic hepatitis C virus infection, cryoglobulins are probably a combination of viral components and certain antibodies against the virus. The cryoglobulins can deposit in the kidney and cause them to malfunction.

As mentioned above, the CBC can tell a lot of things about a person's overall state of health. Some patients with cirrhosis become anemic and have low white blood cell counts. They may also have low platelet counts. Low blood counts can occur, however, as a result of many other conditions.

Patients with cirrhosis as a result of chronic hepatitis C may have abnormalities in their electrolytes (the minerals dissolved in the blood). An electrolyte abnormality sometimes seen in advanced cirrhosis is a low blood sodium, or *hyponatremia*. The blood electrolytes, which include the sodium, potassium, chloride, and bicarbonate concentrations, should be followed carefully in individuals with advanced cirrhosis. Drugs used to treat the complications of cirrhosis may also affect the blood electrolyte concentrations.

Radiological Testing

Radiological tests may be used in the evaluation of patients with liver diseases. Many doctors routinely use a vast array of radiological tests to evaluate patients with chronic hepatitis C. Very frankly, a lot of this testing is *not* medically appropriate. Some radiological scans may be used for the evaluation of complications of chronic hepatitis, such as advanced cirrhosis and liver cancer. Some are appropriate to evaluate other liver diseases. Each of the radiological tests used to evaluate the liver has certain strengths and all have limitations. Following are the most common radiological procedures used in the evaluation of liver diseases:

- Ultrasound or sonography
- Computerized axial tomography scan (CAT scan or CT scan)

- Magnetic resonance imaging (MRI) scan
- Liver–spleen scan
- Tagged red blood cell scan

The reasons for performing these tests and their indications in chronic hepatitis C, if any, are discussed below.

Ultrasound or Sonography

The ultrasound examination or sonogram is the most widely used radiological procedure to evaluate patients with liver diseases. The test is noninvasive and relatively cheap. In most cases of hepatitis C, however, the ultrasound provides no useful information. Nonetheless, most doctors will perform ultrasounds on most patients with chronic hepatitis C.

To perform an ultrasound examination, probes that emit and detect sound waves are placed against the surface of the abdomen. An image based on the deflection and penetration of sound waves is then generated. There are virtually no risks to performing an ultrasound examination of the liver, except incorrect interpretation of the results.

Ultrasound is an excellent test for the detection of liver masses such as tumors or cysts. It is also a powerful method to look for widening of the bile ducts that can result from obstruction by a stone or tumor. The ultrasound provides a clear image of the gallbladder and is very sensitive for detecting gallstones. Combined with another type of sound wave analysis that detects Doppler shifts (a change in the pitch of a sound wave emanating or reflected from a moving object), ultrasound can also provide information about blood flow in the major veins and arteries of the liver.

Ultrasound *cannot* diagnose hepatitis C or accurately assess the degree of inflammation or scar tissue (fibrosis) in the livers of patients with hepatitis C. Ultrasound *cannot* detect early cirrhosis and can only suggest the presence of cirrhosis if it is advanced and the liver is shrunken and nodular. The results of ultrasound scanning provide *no* information about liver function.

Many patients with chronic hepatitis C read their ultrasound test results, thinking that they say something important about the disease. They are concerned about terms such as *echogenic, hetero-geneous*, and *parenchyma. Don't worry about these readings*. These terms, which radiologists use to describe what they see, often tell little, if anything, about the condition of the liver or the disease process. In summary, ultrasound is *not* a primary tool to establish the diagnosis or determine the prognosis in chronic hepatitis C.

Computerized Axial Tomography (CAT or CT)

Computerized axial tomography, better known as CAT or CT scanning, generates an image based on x-rays taken from multiple angles. A patient undergoing a CAT scan lies in a scanner that looks like a giant donut. x-rays are emitted and detected from multiple locations around the body. A computer reconstructs an image based on the penetration and scattering of the x-rays. A CAT scan is a generally safe procedure; one of the few side effects is an allergic reaction to the intravenous contrast dye frequently given to improve the images. Intravenous contrast agents can also cause acute kidney failure in individuals with kidney problems.

CAT scanning of the liver is *not* indicated for the diagnosis or evaluation of a patient with chronic hepatitis C. It should only be used if there is a specific indication to look for something else. If your doctor orders a CAT scan as part of the *routine* evaluation or diagnosis of chronic hepatitis C, ask why! CAT scans *cannot* assess the degree of fibrosis or inflammation in hepatitis C, nor can they establish a diagnosis of hepatitis C. Like ultrasound, CAT scanning can only establish the diagnosis of cirrhosis if it is advanced and the liver is shrunken and nodular. CAT scans can be used to assess tumors or masses in the liver. They should *not* be performed for routine screening for tumors; ultrasound is safer, cheaper, and probably just as effective. CAT scans of the liver are reserved for special indications and are not used to evaluate the majority of patients with chronic hepatitis C.

Magnetic Resonance Imaging

Magnetic resonance imaging (MRI) uses nuclear magnetic resonance to produce images. The patient is placed in a very strong magnetic field to align the spins of the protons in the atoms in the patient's body. Spin relaxation times, the time it takes the protons to change rotation when the body is pulsed with radio waves, are measured and used to generate images of the internal organs. A patient undergoing an MRI scan is usually placed in a small tunnel surrounded by giant magnets. MRI is similar to a CAT scan in its strengths and limitations. It may be slightly more sensitive for the evaluation of certain tumors. It is absolutely not indicated for the diagnosis or the routine evaluation of patients with hepatitis C.

Liver–Spleen Scan

The liver–spleen scan is a nuclear medicine test that can sometimes detect the presence of cirrhosis. In this test, a radioactive compound is injected into the patient and a picture is taken with a camera that detects the emitted radiation. If blood flow to the liver is backed up (portal hypertension), as it could be in cirrhosis, the test will detect a colloid shift in which more of the radioactive material is taken up by the bone marrow as opposed to the liver. The liver–spleen scan is used less often these days and provides useful information in only occasional cases. Some doctors may order it to determine the presence of portal hypertension if cirrhosis is suspected on clinical grounds. It cannot diagnose early cirrhosis.

Tagged Red Blood Cell Scan

In a tagged red blood cell scan, a radioactive material is attached to red blood cells that are then injected into the patient's vein. A picture of the liver is taken with a camera that detects the emitted radioactivity. This test is excellent for detecting *hemangioma*, a common benign vascular tumor of the liver. Because the hemangioma has a very rich blood supply, the radioactive tagged red blood cells accumulate in it. It may be used in a patient with hepatitis C in whom an ultrasound has detected a mass suspected to be a hemangioma.

Liver Biopsy

Liver biopsy plays an important role in the evaluation of a patient with chronic hepatitis C. Unlike the numerous blood tests and radiological procedures to assess the liver, biopsy provides critical information that none of these tests can. With regard to chronic hepatitis C, a liver biopsy is the only way to establish the extent of inflammation and fibrosis (scar tissue) and, in most cases, the presence or absence of cirrhosis. It is also usually the only way to determine if other conditions, such as alcohol consumption or fatty liver, are simultaneously contributing to liver damage. In addition, intelligent decisions regarding appropriate treatment and follow-up for the patient with chronic hepatitis C can generally only be made after examining the liver biopsy.

Performing a Liver Biopsy

In a liver biopsy, a small piece of liver tissue is obtained. This tissue is cut into thin sections and stained with various dyes, usually hematoxylin and eosin, which label different cells and different parts of the cells in various colors. Sometimes special stains for scar tissue or fat are also used. The pathologist, preferably together with the patient's doctor, examines the stained tissue under a microscope to confirm the diagnosis (or various diagnoses), the extent of inflammation, the degree of fibrosis, and the presence or absence of cirrhosis.

Most liver biopsies are performed percutaneously (through the skin) and blindly (without directly visualizing the liver) using a small needle. Liver biopsies can also be performed under ultrasound or CAT scan guidance; however, these approaches should only be used if the doctor is interested in obtaining tissue from a specific area within the liver, for example, from something suspected of being a tumor. Liver biopsies can also be performed using a laparoscope, which is a fiber-optic tube inserted into the abdomen through which the doctor can see the inside of the abdomen and the liver. Laparoscopic liver biopsy should also only be performed for biopsy of a specific abnormality such as a tumor or possibly when the risk of

bleeding from a blind, percutaneous biopsy is increased. Liver biopsies can also be performed via a transjugular approach in which a
catheter is inserted into a vein in the neck and passed to the liver.
The transjugular approach is used only when the patient has a high
risk of bleeding. Liver biopsies can also be performed at surgery.

Unless the risk of bleeding is increased, or a piece of tissue from
a particular mass or tumor is desired, a percutaneous liver biopsy
should generally be performed. This is the case for most patients
with chronic hepatitis C who do not have advanced cirrhosis or a
suspected tumor in the liver. During this procedure, the patient is
awake and not sedated. A percutaneous liver biopsy does *not* hurt
that much. While the patient lies on his or her back, the doctor iden-
tifies a point in a line drawn roughly on the right side from the
armpit to the hip between two ribs (see Figure 4.1). The area is
cleaned with an antiseptic solution and numbed with lidocaine, similar to how a dentist numbs the mouth before filling a cavity. The
doctor breaks the tough surface skin with a sharp metal stick. A
needle at the end of a syringe is placed lightly into the small hole in
the skin. While the patient is breathing calmly, the doctor rapidly
sticks the needle into the liver and withdraws it in one swift motion
that takes less than a second. In the process, a tiny piece of liver is
sucked into the needle attached to the syringe. After the biopsy, the
patient remains in bed for about four hours before being sent home.
During this time, a nurse periodically checks the patient's pulse and
blood pressure to make sure that there is no serious bleeding. I usually do liver biopsies around 8 or 9 A.M., let the patient have lunch
in bed around noon, and send the patient home around 1 or 2 P.M.

The thought of a liver biopsy often provokes considerable anxiety for the patient and also for some doctors. If patients relax
throughout the procedure, the risks are fairly low and there is very
little pain. Many patients equate the sensation of being stuck with
a needle with being punched in the ribs. There may also be some dull
pain in the right shoulder after the biopsy, a referred pain caused by
irritation to the liver capsule. There is usually some bleeding at the
site of the biopsy but not more than can be wiped away with a piece
of cotton. After the biopsy, the doctor will generally put a pressure
dressing over the area to stop the bleeding.

Figure 4.1 A Percutaneous Needle Biopsy of the Liver

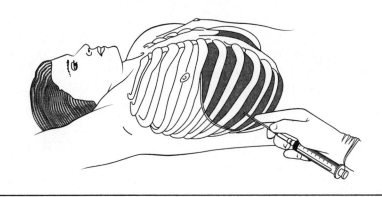

In patients with liver disease who do not have low platelet counts or elevated prothrombin times, percutaneous biopsy is a generally safe procedure. The pain is not severe and goes away after several hours to a day. Acetaminophen (Tylenol) is safe and usually effective in relieving the pain. The major complication of liver biopsy is bleeding that requires blood transfusion or surgery, but this happens in fewer than 1 in 1,000 cases. Punctures of the lung, gallbladder, or intestine, which usually heal themselves, also rarely occur. Although deaths from percutaneous biopsy do occur, they are very rare in patients with normal platelet counts and prothrombin times and the absence of advanced cirrhosis. Prior to doing a liver biopsy, the doctor should check the patient's complete blood count, especially the platelet count, and the prothrombin time.

If the platelet count is too low, the prothrombin time too high, or significant ascites (fluid in the abdomen) is present, a percutaneous liver biopsy should probably not be performed. In these cases, liver tissue can be obtained by the transjugular or laparoscopic approaches. An open surgical liver biopsy can be performed if all other approaches are determined to be too risky or are unsuccessful (this is rarely the case). Blind, percutaneous biopsy is usually not appropriate if the aim is to obtain tissue from a liver tumor. In such cases, a biopsy should be performed by a radiologist under ultrasound or CAT scan guidance, with a laparoscope, or by a surgeon in an open procedure.

What Does a Liver Biopsy Tell in a Case of Chronic Hepatitis C?

The biopsy is examined for several reasons: to confirm the diagnosis of chronic hepatitis C, to include or exclude other problems, to assess the degree of inflammation, to assess the extent of fibrosis (scar tissue), and to determine if the liver is cirrhotic. In most cases, reasonable decisions about prognosis and treatment can only be made after a liver biopsy is performed.

A liver biopsy is important and usually indicated in patients with chronic hepatitis C for the following reasons:

A liver biopsy is used to confirm the diagnosis of chronic hepatitis C. Rarely can a pathologist look at a liver biopsy alone and say that it is definitely hepatitis C. Liver inflammation in hepatitis C often looks like liver inflammation in other forms of hepatitis, such as that caused by the hepatitis B virus, some drugs, and some metabolic diseases. There are some features, however, that can make a pathologist pretty certain that the liver disease is hepatitis C just by looking at the biopsy. What is important is that, given the history of infection with the hepatitis C virus, the observed abnormalities on the liver biopsy are consistent with those that the virus are known to cause.

A liver biopsy can establish the presence of other liver diseases besides chronic hepatitis C. Individuals with hepatitis C may drink excessive amounts of alcohol or may have other relatively common liver diseases, such as hemochromatosis, drug hepatitis, or fatty liver. A liver biopsy can help determine how much the hepatitis C virus itself is contributing to liver damage and how much is caused by other factors.

A liver biopsy is the only way to accurately assess the degree of inflammation. Chronic hepatitis C is characterized by the presence of significantly abnormal numbers of inflammatory cells (white blood cells known as lymphocytes) invading the liver. By examining the biopsy, the pathologist can say something about the extent of inflammation. Sometimes, the pathologist will describe the inflammation as mild, moderate, or severe. Often, the degree of inflammation is given a numerical grade with 0 being no inflammation and 3 being severe. In some research studies, more complex numerical scores are given for the degree of inflammation. It is important to emphasize that, at the present time, no test except a liver biopsy can accurately assess the degree of liver inflammation in hepatitis C (or any type of hepatitis). Blood aminotransferase activities do *not* precisely correlate with the degree of liver inflammation.

A liver biopsy is the only way to accurately assess the degree of fibrosis in the liver. Chronic liver inflammation in hepatitis C results in the formation of fibrosis or scar tissue. In some cases, there may be no or very little fibrosis after many decades of infection. In other cases, there may be marked fibrosis and even cirrhosis. No blood test or radiological test can accurately determine the degree of liver fibrosis in a patient with chronic hepatitis C. Therefore, a liver biopsy is essential to assess the degree of fibrosis. This information may be the most important of all for someone with chronic hepatitis C. Significant fibrosis suggests that cirrhosis will likely develop in the future. Some pathologists give a numerical stage to the degree of fibrosis, with 0 being none and 4 being cirrhosis. A score of 3 indicates bridging fibrosis, a type of scarring that starts to develop into cirrhosis. In some research studies, more complicated scoring systems may be used to describe the degree of liver fibrosis.

A liver biopsy is the only way to diagnose cirrhosis in most patients with chronic hepatitis C, or any other chronic liver disease. Some patients with chronic hepatitis C will seek medical attention only when they have obvious clinical complications of cirrhosis, such as jaundice (yellow skin), ascites (fluid in the abdomen), encephalopathy (mental confusion), or bleeding from ruptured varicose veins in the esophagus. However, cirrhosis is frequently present prior to the development of symptoms. In such instances, cirrhosis can only be diagnosed by a liver biopsy. This is true for most individuals with cirrhosis caused by chronic hepatitis.

Anatomically, cirrhosis is defined by the presence of fibrosis and widespread nodules in the liver. Fibrosis is scar tissue that likely results from a long period of inflammation and liver cell death. Nodules are abnormally regenerating clusters of liver cells. In many cases, the presence of extensive fibrosis and regenerating nodules (cirrhosis) can only be established by microscopic examination of liver tissue. This is why a liver biopsy is often necessary in chronic hepatitis C.

A liver biopsy is often the only way to obtain reliable information about prognosis and treatment in chronic hepatitis C. Individuals with hepatitis C and cirrhosis have a worse prognosis than those who do not have cirrhosis. Cirrhosis is the outcome to be avoided in chronic hepatitis C; nearly all serious and life-threatening aspects of chronic hepatitis C result from the development of cirrhosis. A patient can have chronic hepatitis C for his or her entire life. If he or she does not develop cirrhosis, it is extremely unlikely that the disease will affect the quality of life or life expectancy in any way. In advanced cirrhosis, the liver becomes shrunken and very nodular. As cirrhosis becomes more severe, the liver begins to fail and complications ensue (see Chapter 5). Cirrhosis is also associated with the development of liver cancer, which rarely occurs in hepatitis C in the absence of cirrhosis. Early cirrhosis can only be diagnosed by liver biopsy.

The degree of inflammation and fibrosis evident in a liver biopsy tells something about the chance of developing cirrhosis. Individuals with chronic hepatitis C with significant degrees of fibrosis and inflammation in a liver biopsy are more likely than those with minimal to no inflammation and fibrosis to go on to develop cirrhosis. Individuals who already have significant fibrosis or significant inflammation should probably consider undergoing treatment sooner rather than later, as they are more likely to progress to cirrhosis, the complication we hope to prevent. Individuals who have had hepatitis C virus infection for many years but have minimal to no inflammation or fibrosis may be more willing to wait a few years to see if better treatments become available, or possibly decide not to be treated at all. In short, logical advice regarding prognosis and treatment can usually only be given to the patient with chronic hepatitis C after a liver biopsy is examined.

When a Liver Biopsy Is Not Recommended

Liver biopsy is *not* indicated for everyone. Examples include:

- In a patient with clinically advanced cirrhosis and clinical complications, the liver biopsy usually provides little additional information. If the presence of cirrhosis with complications can be established on clinical grounds, there is little reason to do a liver biopsy to establish the degree of inflammation or fibrosis. There is generally little to offer a patient with hepatitis C and complications of cirrhosis in the way of treatment, except to manage the complications and refer the patient for liver transplantation if and when it is appropriate. A patient with advanced cirrhosis may sometimes require liver biopsy when it is not clear if another undiagnosed disease (besides or in addition to hepatitis C) is part of the problem.
- In patients with hepatitis C and concurrent diseases more immediately serious and life threatening, the biopsy can sometimes be deferred until the other diseases are under

control. For example, you would *not* do a liver biopsy on someone with hepatitis C who just had a heart attack or someone with cancer that may be terminal and untreatable. In some cases, a patient may have a much more serious illness than hepatitis C.

- Some patients have medical problems in which the risks of liver biopsy outweigh the benefits. A patient who has a serious blood-clotting disorder may not be a candidate for liver biopsy.

- Because hepatitis C is a slowly progressive disease, there is usually little reason to do a liver biopsy in an elderly patient who has chronic hepatitis C. For example, if an eighty-year-old person has chronic hepatitis C but is otherwise healthy, there is no reason to further evaluate the extent of liver damage. This person already has a great prognosis and will likely die of other causes before developing complications of cirrhosis.

The decision whether or not to do a liver biopsy in a patient with chronic hepatitis C depends on the judgment of an *experienced* doctor. In general, most patients with chronic hepatitis C who are relatively young and do not have other serious diseases or complications of cirrhosis should probably have a liver biopsy. Patients who are elderly or have other serious health problems probably should not. I again stress that a physician with experience in caring for patients with liver diseases should make the final decision about a liver biopsy in a patient with chronic hepatitis C.

5

Prognosis of Chronic Hepatitis C

CIRRHOSIS IS THE dreaded complication of chronic hepatitis C. Some individuals with cirrhosis can survive to a ripe old age without suffering complications, but most of the serious and life-threatening aspects of chronic hepatitis C result from cirrhosis. The complications of cirrhosis can kill or necessitate liver transplantation. In the United States, cirrhosis from chronic hepatitis C is the number one indication for liver transplantation. (There is more cirrhosis from alcohol, but active alcohol abusers generally do not receive liver transplants.) A liver affected by both hepatitis C and cirrhosis is also more likely to develop cancer than a liver with hepatitis C and no cirrhosis.

The first part of this chapter discusses in detail cirrhosis and its complications. But remember: *Most people with chronic hepatitis C will not develop complications of cirrhosis and will live long lives and die of something else.*

Cirrhosis and Its Complications

Many people associate the term *cirrhosis* only with excessive alcohol consumption. In the United States, alcohol abuse is indeed the leading cause of cirrhosis, though virtually any chronic liver disease can cause it. *In the United States, the number two cause of cirrhosis is chronic hepatitis C.* Individuals with chronic hepatitis C who also abuse alcohol have a greatly enhanced risk of developing cirrhosis.

Anatomically, fibrosis and widespread nodules in the liver characterize cirrhosis. Fibrosis is the deposition of scar tissue. Nodules form as dying liver cells are replaced by regenerating ones. Unfortunately, this regeneration results in an abnormal liver architecture.

In early stages, the nodules and fibrosis may only be detected by microscopic examination of liver tissue obtained by biopsy. The patient may have no symptoms and live a normal, sometimes very active life. Ultimately, the fibrosis and nodule formation in cirrhosis causes distortion of the liver's architecture, which interferes with blood flow through the organ. Cirrhosis can also lead to an inability of the liver to perform its major biochemical functions. As cirrhosis becomes more advanced, the abnormalities in the liver's blood flow and biochemical functions lead to several potentially serious complications. These problems can lead to morbidity of the liver and the need for liver transplantation to survive. The major complications of cirrhosis are listed below:

- Splenomegaly (enlarged spleen)
- Bleeding from esophageal and gastric varices (varicose veins)
- Edema (generalized fluid retention)
- Ascites (edema in the abdomen)
- Jaundice (yellow discoloration of skin from bilirubin retention)
- Hepatic encephalopathy (mental changes ranging from mild confusion to coma)
- Bleeding tendencies
- Low or high blood sugars
- Increased susceptibility to infections
- Spontaneous bacterial peritonitis (infected fluid in abdomen)
- Kidney failure (including hepatorenal syndrome)
- Generalized muscle wasting
- Hyponatremia (low blood sodium concentration)

Portal Hypertension

In cirrhosis, blood flow through the liver is impeded because of the liver's abnormal architecture. As a result, blood backs up in the portal vein, a major vessel that delivers blood to the liver. This leads to elevated blood pressure in the portal circulation—the circulation of the gut—known as *portal hypertension*. Portal hypertension sometimes occurs in severe cases of acute hepatitis and other forms of liver damage, but cirrhosis is by far the leading cause. Portal hypertension can cause several serious problems including *splenomegaly* and *esophageal* and *gastric varices*.

Splenomegaly

Because the portal vein is connected to the splenic vein, portal hypertension can cause blood to back up in the spleen. This causes the spleen to become enlarged and trap blood cells, a condition known as *splenomegaly*. Sequestration of platelets in an abnormally enlarged spleen can cause a drop in the platelet count and abnormal bleeding tendencies.

Esophageal and Gastric Varices

As the pressure in the portal circulation increases, blood can flow backward into the systemic venous circulation at certain points where they are connected. Prominent connections between the portal and systemic venous circulations occur in the esophagus and the stomach. Portal hypertension can lead to varicose veins in the stomach and esophagus, known as *gastric* and *esophageal varices*. The portal and systemic circulations are also connected in the rectum, where increased portal pressure can cause hemorrhoids. The two circulations also connect under the skin in the abdomen and increased pressure can cause a group of veins to visibly congest and swell, called a *caput medusa*.

Gastric and esophageal varices are among the most serious complications of portal hypertension because they can rupture and bleed. Internal bleeding from esophageal and gastric varices can be massive and life threatening. The patient will often experience nausea and vomiting when gastric or esophageal varices bleed. The vomit usually has a "coffee ground" appearance, which results from the action of stomach acid on blood: The acid causes clumps of normally soluble material to denature and fall out of solution, hence the blood looks like coffee grounds. Bleeding gastric and esophageal varices can also cause black, tarry stools known as *melana* if partially digested blood passes through the digestive tract. Patients with either coffee ground emesis (vomit) or melana (black stools) should head immediately to the emergency room, as these symptoms are a result of internal bleeding in the upper gastrointestinal tract.

Edema and Ascites

Hypertension in the portal circulation, along with complex hormonal, metabolic, and possibly kidney abnormalities in cirrhosis, can lead to fluid accumulation. *Edema* is the general term for fluid retention in the body. In cirrhosis, there is a tendency for the abdomen to retain fluid. Abnormal fluid in the abdomen is called *ascites*. In cirrhosis, ascites may not be present or may be massive (gallons of fluid). It is not uncommon for a patient with cirrhosis to first seek medical attention because he or she can no longer fit into a pair of pants or a dress. Because of the tendency to retain fluid, patients with cirrhosis should have their weight checked periodically.

Jaundice

Bilirubin is taken up by the healthy liver, conjugated to a more water-soluble form, and secreted into the bile. In cirrhosis, there is decreased bilirubin secretion from hepatocytes into the bile. This leads to the backup of bilirubin in the blood, elevated blood bilirubin concentrations, and jaundice. As the conjugated form of bilirubin backs up in the blood, bilirubin can spill into the urine, giving it a bright yellow to dark brown color. The increased concentration of bilirubin in the blood causes people with advanced liver disease to appear yellow.

Hepatic Encephalopathy

Hepatic encephalopathy is abnormal brain function, ranging from subtle changes in mental status to deep coma, that occurs when the liver fails. Hepatic encephalopathy can occur in advanced cirrhosis. In cirrhosis, blood laden with metabolic by-products and toxins leaving the gut bypasses the liver hepatocytes as a result of the abnormal architecture. Metabolism of certain compounds absorbed in the gut may also be decreased within the liver as biochemical function deteriorates. Both of these derangements can lead to hepatic encephalopathy as toxic metabolites, normally removed from the blood by the liver, reach the brain.

In its early stages, hepatic encephalopathy is characterized by subtle mental changes, such as poor concentration or irritability. One of the first problems is the inability to construct simple objects such as a six-point star out of toothpicks. Another early sign is difficulty with connect-the-dot drawings. Various degrees of confusion and sleepiness occur in more advanced cases. In severe cases, the patient falls into a stupor or coma and eventually dies.

Infectious Complications

Individuals with cirrhosis may have depressed immune systems and be at a higher risk for more types of infections than healthy individuals. One infectious complication unique to individuals with ascites is *spontaneous bacterial peritonitis* (SBP). In SBP, the fluid retained in the abdomen becomes spontaneously infected with the bacteria present in the colon. If not adequately treated with antibiotics, SBP can lead to sepsis, an overwhelming infection of the blood, and death.

Other Complications

Cachexia

Patients with cirrhosis have generalized wasting, known as *cachexia*. In advanced cirrhosis, there is significant loss of muscle mass even if nutrient intake is maintained. This loss is usually most noticeable in the temporal muscles on the sides of the head just in front of the ears. Patients with end-stage cirrhosis and ascites often look like balloons with toothpicks for arms and legs, as fluid accumulates in the abdomen and muscle mass is lost in the extremities.

It is not entirely understood why muscle wasting occurs in patients with cirrhosis and some other chronic diseases. It may result in part from the abnormal production of various *cytokines*, compounds secreted into the blood that alter body metabolism. As a result, patients develop an overall metabolic state in which muscle proteins are degraded more rapidly than they are synthesized. Patients with cirrhosis usually have high circulating levels of the *cytokine tumor necrosis factor*, or *cachexin*, which causes wasting when injected into animals.

Bleeding Tendencies

In cirrhosis, the platelet counts fall secondary to abnormal trapping of platelets in an enlarged spleen. The prothrombin time is also increased as a result of decreased synthesis of certain blood-clotting factors in the failing liver. As a result of these alterations, individuals with cirrhosis have an increased chance of bleeding. Decreased blood-clotting capability can be a major aggravating factor in patients with gastric or esophageal varices that rupture and bleed, as the chances of stopping the bleeding decrease.

Electrolyte Abnormalities

Abnormalities in total body fluid balance and altered kidney and hormone function in cirrhosis can lead to problems with blood electrolytes. Electrolytes are soluble mineral elements in the form of ions in the blood. The most abundant electrolytes in the blood are sodium and chloride (table salt). Bicarbonate and potassium are also important blood electrolytes. Significant abnormalities in their concentrations can result in numerous problems.

The electrolyte abnormality most often seen in advanced cirrhosis, especially in patients with edema and ascites, is *hyponatremia,* an abnormally low sodium concentration in the blood. Severe hyponatremia can cause seizures and other brain abnormalities. Although the sodium concentration may be low in the blood, the total body sodium paradoxically *increases* in patients with cirrhosis and hyponatremia. Administration of excess sodium only worsens the problem by increasing the amount of ascites and edema.

As patients with cirrhosis and ascites may have subtle kidney abnormalities and are often thirsty secondary to hormonal changes, drinking of excess water contributes to hyponatremia. Hyponatremia will generally improve if water intake is restricted. In very severe cases of hyponatremia, intravenous administration of concentrated sodium solutions may be necessary to prevent seizures, even though this may worsen ascites and edema. This must be done slowly and carefully and only in a hospital with very close monitoring.

Kidney Abnormalities

Cirrhosis leads to abnormalities in kidney function, which range from mild to complete kidney shutdown. Subtle alterations in kidney function and consequent hormonal changes contribute to the formation of ascites and edema and the development of hyponatremia. In advanced cases of cirrhosis, a type of kidney failure known as *hepatorenal syndrome* can occur. In hepatorenal syndrome, for unclear reasons, the kidneys fail to function. Surprisingly, the same kidneys work fine if they are transplanted into a normal body; for some reason, advanced cirrhosis makes them shut down. Hepatorenal syndrome can be treated with dialysis for a short time; however, it is virtually always fatal unless liver transplantation is performed. If the liver is replaced, kidney function returns to normal.

Other Metabolic Complications

There are several other metabolic complications associated with cirrhosis.

- Albumin concentration in the blood decreases, which can enhance the formation of ascites and edema.
- The metabolism of many drugs is decreased and the dosages of some medications must be appropriately adjusted.
- In men, breast enlargement or *gynecomastia* sometimes occurs because metabolism of estrogens by the liver is decreased. Atrophy of the testicles can also occur.

- Derangements in the metabolism of triglycerides and cholesterol can occur. Usually, the blood cholesterol concentration is very low, except in cases of cirrhosis caused by bile duct obstruction where it can be abnormally elevated.
- In the early stages of cirrhosis, insulin resistance can develop, which leads to high blood sugar. In advanced stages of cirrhosis, blood sugar may be dangerously low because it cannot be synthesized from glycogen, fats, or proteins in the failing liver.

Liver Cancer

Cirrhosis from any cause increases the risk of developing *hepatocellular carcinoma*, a primary liver cancer. Hepatocellular carcinoma is fairly rare in the Western hemisphere; however, in East Asia, primarily because of the high prevalence of chronic viral hepatitis, hepatocellular carcinoma is the number one or number two cause of cancer death. Although patients with chronic hepatitis C without cirrhosis occasionally develop hepatocellular carcinoma, most cases occur in cirrhotic livers. It is not entirely clear why cirrhosis increases the risk of developing liver cancer. It undoubtedly has something to do with the abnormal regeneration of cells. The hepatitis C virus may slightly predispose cells to become cancerous. Abnormal-looking or dysplastic cells in cirrhotic livers can look precancerous; presumably, these cells can eventually become cancerous and form tumors.

There is not much that can be done to prevent the development of cancer in a cirrhotic liver except monitoring. About 80 percent of hepatocellular carcinomas make a protein known as alpha-fetoprotein, which is secreted into the blood. Occasional blood tests that screen blood alpha-fetoprotein concentration are a reasonable method for detecting early liver cancer in patients with cirrhosis. However, blood alpha-fetoprotein may sometimes be slightly elevated in the absence of cancer, and not all hepatocellular carcinomas elevate blood alpha-fetoprotein. Periodic ultrasound screening is another method for detecting cancer, but the efficacy of these screenings to detect hepatocellular carcinoma in a patient with cirrhosis and hepatitis C is not firmly established. Some studies from Asian countries (where cirrhosis results mostly from chronic hepatitis B) suggest that annual or biannual screenings may be effective in detecting early, potentially treatable cancers. Most doctors in the United States will probably screen a patient with chronic hepatitis C and cirrhosis once a year; others do it every six months.

Diagnosis of Cirrhosis

Cirrhosis is usually an easy diagnosis when some or all of the above complications are present in a chronically ill individual with a history of liver disease. Virtually any chronic liver disease can cause cirrhosis. Some conditions can mimic various signs and symptoms of cirrhosis. These include abdominal cancers, clots in the hepatic or portal veins that respectively exit and enter the liver, severe acute hepatitis, congestive heart failure, and pericaditis, or swelling around the heart. A careful history, combined with special diagnostic tests, will usually identify these conditions.

As emphasized in previous chapters, some individuals with cirrhosis, especially early in the course of the disease, will have *no* overt clinical signs or symptoms. Radiological and nuclear medicine tests will only suggest the presence of cirrhosis in fairly advanced cases. In most patients without clinical complications, the diagnosis of cirrhosis usually requires a liver biopsy (see Chapter 4).

Will I Develop Cirrhosis and Its Complications?

For most individuals, the scariest part of suffering from chronic hepatitis C is the constant question "Will I develop cirrhosis and its complications?" The big problem for patients and doctors is that the prognosis of chronic hepatitis C is extremely variable and often cannot be accurately predicted in a specific case. Many patients, perhaps most, will have mild, low-grade hepatitis for life and *never* develop cirrhosis and its complications. Some patients will develop cirrhosis several years after infection. Some will not have symptoms for many years, then see a doctor later in life with clinical evidence of cirrhosis. Many people will never even know that they are infected with the hepatitis C virus. A few hypothetical case histories are illustrative.

Patient 1

An eighty-four-year-old woman has swelling of the abdomen, swollen ankles, and yellowing of her eyes. She has never drunk alcohol. When she was thirty-four, she had a hysterectomy and needed a blood transfusion because of extensive bleeding during surgery. She was an active, healthy woman for the next forty years with few visits to doctors. Physical examination now reveals ascites, edema, and jaundice. Blood testing shows slightly elevated ALT and AST activities, low albumin concentration, elevated bilirubin concentration, and a prolonged prothrombin time. An ultrasound shows ascites and a shrunken, nodular liver consistent with cirrhosis with a mass very typical of hepatocellular carcinoma. A blood test for antibodies against the hepatitis C virus comes back positive, and a PCR test is also positive at 1,000,000 copies per milliliter; the genotype is 1b.

Patient 2

Another eighty-four-year-old woman is followed by a doctor for high blood pressure and diabetes mellitus but is otherwise healthy. When she was thirty-four, she had a hysterectomy and needed a blood transfusion because of extensive bleeding during surgery. Except for high blood pressure and diabetes, which are treated with medications, she has been in excellent health. On routine blood testing, her ALT is found to be slightly elevated. Looking back over many years, her ALT had been normal on most occasions and mildly elevated a couple of times. Albumin, bilirubin, and prothrombin time are normal. A test for antibodies against the hepatitis C virus comes back positive, and a PCR test is also positive at 1,000,000 copies per milliliter; the genotype is 1b.

Patient 3

A fifty-year-old woman has progressive swelling of the abdomen, swollen ankles, and yellowing of her eyes. She has never drunk alcohol. When she was thirty-four, she had a hysterectomy and needed a blood transfusion because of extensive bleeding during surgery. She was an active, healthy woman for the next twelve years with few visits to doctors. For the past four years, she has had increasing fatigue and gradually increasing swelling in the ankles and abdomen. Physical examination now reveals ascites, edema, and jaundice. Blood testing shows slightly elevated ALT and AST activities, low albumin concentration, elevated bilirubin concentration, and a prolonged prothrombin time. An ultrasound shows ascites and a shrunken, nodular liver consistent with cirrhosis. A blood test for antibodies against the hepatitis C virus comes back positive, and a PCR test is also positive at 1,000,000 copies per milliliter; the genotype is 1b. A transjugular liver biopsy is consistent with chronic hepatitis C and cirrhosis.

These three hypothetical patients illustrate the highly variable course of chronic hepatitis C. Patients 1 and 2, both now eighty-four years old, were both infected with the hepatitis C virus at age thirty-four by blood transfusion. Neither drank alcohol and both were healthy most of their lives. After fifty years of infection, patient 1 has developed cirrhosis and liver cancer, while patient 2 has no significant liver disease. Both have lived to a nice old age. Patient 1 will probably die from complications of liver disease. Patient 2 will probably live several more years and die of another cause, perhaps heart disease as a complication of diabetes and high blood pressure. Patient 3, on the other hand, demonstrates a fairly rapid development of cirrhosis. She, too, was infected with the hepatitis C virus at age thirty-four and developed complications of cirrhosis in about fifteen years. She will probably receive a liver transplant in her fifties. It is not clear from these histories why patient 1 developed serious liver disease in fifty years, why patient 2 has no significant liver disease after fifty years, and why patient 3 developed serious liver disease after only fifteen years of hepatitis C virus infection.

Let us look at three similar cases in a different way. Three forty-four-year-old women see their doctors because they had slightly elevated ALT activities on blood testing as part of life insurance examinations. All three had received blood transfusions at age thirty-four because of complications from surgical hysterectomies. All three are found to have antibodies against the hepatitis C virus. All three are otherwise healthy. Which one may have complications of cirrhosis in five years? Which one will live another fifty years and never develop significant liver disease? Which one may develop significant liver disease in another fifty years? There is no way to say for sure; however, some further testing may give the doctors clues.

The best test to obtain prognostic information about chronic hepatitis C infection in a patient who does not have obvious complications of cirrhosis is a liver biopsy. As discussed previously, a liver biopsy can establish the degree of inflammation, the degree of fibrosis, and the presence or absence of cirrhosis. Patients with significant inflammation and fibrosis are more likely to develop cirrhosis than those who do not have fibrosis or have only minimal fibrosis. Patients whose biopsy indicates cirrhosis are at a much greater risk for developing complications, liver failure, and hepatocellular carcinoma.

For example, if one of these three hypothetical forty-four-year-old women had cirrhosis in a liver biopsy and the other two did not, she would have a greater chance of developing complications of cirrhosis in the next several years. However, it would still be impossible to predict precisely when complications of cirrhosis would arise, or if she would live with cirrhosis for many years and never develop serious complications. If one of the three women had absolutely no inflammation and no fibrosis in a liver biopsy, there would be a good chance that she would live many years and never develop significant liver disease (like patient 2 discussed previously). However, it would also be possible that she would develop cirrhosis and clinical liver disease after many years (like patient 1 discussed previously). In short, the biopsy gives predictive, but not definitive, information about prognosis in patients with chronic hepatitis C.

Excessive alcohol consumption is an important cofactor for liver damage in patients with chronic hepatitis C. If one of the women discussed above drank significant amounts of alcohol, she would have a greater chance of developing cirrhosis and complications. The two following hypothetical patients illustrate this point.

Patient 4

A forty-seven-year-old man arrives at the emergency room drunk, with multiple injuries after a fall. He used intravenous drugs about thirty years ago but has not used them since then. However, for the past thirty years he has continued to drink at least ten beers a day during the week and significantly more on weekends. Blood testing reveals elevated ALT, AST, prothrombin time, and bilirubin concentration. The blood albumin concentration is low. Antibodies against the hepatitis C virus are detected in his blood. A liver biopsy shows cirrhosis. A year later, the patient returns to the emergency room with ascites, jaundice, and hepatic encephalopathy.

Patient 5

A forty-seven-year-old man arrives at the emergency room drunk, with multiple injuries after a fall. Thirty years ago, he drank heavily and used intravenous drugs but has not used intravenous drugs since then. For the past twenty-five years, he has rarely had more than one or two drinks a week. A few times a year he goes on a drinking binge. This weekend he fell and injured himself during one of those binges. Blood testing reveals elevated ALT and AST activities. The bilirubin, albumin, and prothrombin time are normal. Antibodies against the hepatitis C virus are detected in his blood. A liver biopsy shows moderate inflammation and minimal fibrosis. He is considered for treatment for chronic hepatitis C.

Although there may be other differences between patient 4 and patient 5, one major difference is the amount of alcohol they consume. Patient 4, a heavy alcohol consumer with chronic hepatitis C, already had cirrhosis and rapidly developed complications. Patient 5, the moderate binge drinker with chronic hepatitis C, has inflammation and minimal fibrosis and may respond to treatment.

Several independent studies and clinical observations have suggested that alcohol is an independent risk factor for the progression of disease and the development of cirrhosis in individuals with chronic hepatitis C. In fact, the diagnosis of "cirrhosis caused by alcohol *and* hepatitis C" is fairly common on the medical wards these days. Mickey Mantle, the magnificent Yankee baseball player, is perhaps the most famous person who suffered from this combination.

What is not clear about alcohol as a risk factor for the progression of liver disease in patients with hepatitis C is the *amount* of alcohol consumption that increases the risk. Certainly, alcohol consumption of six or more drinks a day will increase the risk of liver disease in any person, but the risk likely increases in individuals with chronic hepatitis C. The data, however, are less clear for lower amounts of alcohol consumption. Most liver specialists agree that more than two alcoholic drinks a day will increase the risk of developing cirrhosis in patients with chronic hepatitis C. Although the precise amounts cannot be established, alcohol consumption will definitely affect the prognosis of a person with hepatitis C.

Viral genotype and concentration of hepatitis C virus RNA in the blood (the viral load) have been considered as predictors of disease progression in chronic hepatitis C. They provide less information than what you see in a liver biopsy. Some studies have shown that infection with hepatitis C virus genotypes 1a or 1b is correlated with a worse prognosis than infection with non–type 1 genotypes. However, there are methodological and design limitations to most published studies that have addressed this issue, and not all studies are in agreement. Even if the association between genotype 1 infection and an increased risk of cirrhosis is true, most patients infected with hepatitis C virus type 1 genotypes will never develop cirrhosis and some with non–type 1 genotypes will. The same holds true for viral loads determined by PCR testing. Patients who have relatively high concentrations of viral RNA in the blood may be more likely to develop cirrhosis than those with lower concentrations.

However, blood viral RNA concentrations can show considerable fluctuation in a given individual, making viral load a very poor predictor of who will and who will not develop cirrhosis. In general, patients infected with type 1 genotypes of the hepatitis C virus with high viral loads *may* have a greater chance of developing cirrhosis than those infected with non–type 1 genotypes and lower viral loads. In short, there is a wide variability, and the viral load is not a good prognostic indicator.

Many factors affect the progression of chronic hepatitis C to cirrhosis. Unfortunately, as demonstrated by hypothetical patients 1, 2, and 3, most of the variables are not known. Patients 1, 2, and 3 are all women infected at the same age with the same genotype of the hepatitis C virus. All had the same viral loads when measured and did not drink alcohol. One went on to develop serious liver disease in fifteen years, one in fifty years, and one not at all. These differences in how the hepatitis C virus affects the liver are likely due to what scientists call host factors: genetic differences in how people respond to infection with the virus. At this time, these genetic factors have not been identified. Just as combinations of many slight genetic differences can make people look dramatically different, combinations of many slight genetic differences make people respond differently to infection with the hepatitis C virus. Future research utilizing the results of the Human Genome Project will hopefully identify host factors that influence a person's response to infection with the hepatitis C virus and lead to the development of tests to better predict a specific person's prognosis. Until then, *examination of the liver biopsy remains the best predictor of prognosis in a patient with chronic hepatitis C.*

Knowledge of the infecting viral genotype may also help predict prognosis. But because there is so much variability, the use of genotype as a good predictor for outcome is questionable. Genotype may be more useful in predicting response to treatment with interferon alpha, as patients infected with type 1 genotypes tend to do less well with treatment. Viral load is not a good prognostic test.

If you look at all patients chronically infected with the hepatitis C virus, how many will develop cirrhosis and possible complications in their lifetimes? This is a big question and the answer is not known. Pharmaceutical companies that manufacture drugs to treat hepatitis C like to throw out a number of about 25 percent. Some retrospective studies of the general population, however, indicate that only a few percent of patients with chronic hepatitis C developed clinically significant liver disease. On the other hand, studies of highly selected patients referred to hospitals specializing in the treatment of liver diseases show that about 50 percent of those with chronic hepatitis C have cirrhosis and some have liver cancer.

In the absence of conclusive data on people infected with the hepatitis C virus, I like to divide infected individuals into three groups. This division is based on some available studies and clinical observations. It helps explain the apparently different rates of progression reported in various studies of patients with chronic hepatitis C.

My first group contains people who are not diagnosed and do not have significant symptoms. In one published study, screening identified sixty healthy blood donors infected with the hepatitis C virus. They all had liver biopsies and only one had evidence of significant liver disease. Most of these patients will probably do very well and never suffer from complications of liver disease. Another study followed a group of pregnant women in Ireland who were treated with contaminated batches of anti-D immune globulin to prevent Rh immunization in 1977 and 1978. Seventeen years after being infected with the hepatitis C virus from the contaminated batches, blood ALT activities were mildly elevated in 47 percent of the subjects. Liver biopsies showed inflammation in 98 percent of cases, with fibrosis in 51 percent. Only two of these women had cirrhosis seventeen years after infection. The average age of these women was forty-five. The big question is, what will their livers look like in another seventeen years, at age sixty-two? My guess is that most will not have cirrhosis and complications of liver disease but that some will. Only a minority of people in this first group with chronic hepatitis C will develop serious liver disease, but it is not always possible to say which people.

My second group of patients with chronic hepatitis C contains people who see doctors for the disease but do not have evidence of serious liver disease. People in this group know they have chronic hepatitis C. Many or most of these patients have had liver biopsies showing inflammation of the liver, fibrosis, developing cirrhosis, or sometimes established cirrhosis without clinical symptoms or complications. Just like my first group, there are no definitive data regarding how many of these patients will develop complications of cirrhosis or serious liver disease over many years. Many investigators estimate that about 25 percent of patients with chronic hepatitis C who are followed by doctors for the disease will develop cirrhosis over twenty or more years. However, there are no definitive data to support this rate. Members of this second group should still be optimistic, as the majority of people who have chronic hepatitis and see doctors will *not* go on to develop complications of cirrhosis in their lifetimes. Nonetheless, as in my first group, it is difficult to predict which individuals will develop problems over many years. This second group will probably benefit most from treatment.

Patients with hepatitis C who do not know they have the disease until they develop complications of cirrhosis comprise my third group. Many of these people see doctors who specialize in liver diseases. Some are sent immediately to liver transplantation centers. These patients are already very sick from chronic hepatitis C, and many or most will ultimately need a liver transplant to survive.

People with chronic hepatitis C can progress from one group to another. As screening becomes more widespread, many people in the first group will enter the second group. Some may go from the first group straight into the third group if they do not see a doctor until they already have serious liver disease. Patients in the second group may move into the third group if their liver disease progresses.

These groups are, of course, artificial constructs; do not take this concept as a scientific classification of patients with chronic hepatitis C. This grouping is meant to help you understand that chronic hepatitis C is a variable disease. Most of the 100 to 170 million people with chronic hepatitis C are in the first group and will *not* die from liver disease. Others with chronic hepatitis C in the United States and developed countries are in the second group and most of them also will *not* die from liver disease. Only a minority of people with the hepatitis C virus are in the third group; however, they still may not die from liver disease. Liver transplantation is a lifesaver of last resort for these individuals. If you have chronic hepatitis C, it is important to remain optimistic about your life. Make long-term plans and assume that you will live a long and complete life!

6

Current Treatment of Hepatitis C and Its Complications

CURRENT TREATMENT OF chronic hepatitis C is based on interferon alpha. Interferon alpha is a reasonably good treatment for hepatitis C, but it is far from perfect. Under the best circumstances, only about half of all patients have the most desired outcome: not having detectable hepatitis C virus in the blood several months after stopping treatment. Interferon alpha causes myriad side effects, including draining the pocketbook. Interferon alpha is not absorbed orally and must be administered by injection. But although interferon alpha is not perfect, it is currently the *only* option available.

Interferon alpha-based treatment for chronic hepatitis C has become more complicated as several pharmaceutical companies have similar competing products. Doctors also use slightly different treatment protocols. The best results are obtained when interferon alpha is combined with ribavirin, an oral antiviral agent, which further complicates treatment regimens. The recent introduction of modified, longer acting versions of interferon alpha has made treatment options even more confusing for patients and doctors alike.

It would be incredibly boring to provide every detail on all the dosages and possible treatment protocols involving interferon alpha that are now used to treat chronic hepatitis C. I instead review the drugs that are currently or will soon be approved in the United States and emphasize what are generally considered the best options. The major side effects of treatment and the retreatment options for those who have had an unsuccessful first course are summarized. I also provide some thoughts on who should and should not be treated, realizing that the decision in a specific case must be left to the individual patient and his or her doctor. In Chapter 9, potentially better treatments for chronic hepatitis C that may be available in the future are discussed.

When reading these sections please remember this: *Treatment decisions and recommendations in a specific case can only be made by a doctor who examines the patient and knows his or her complete history.* No one treatment is suitable for all patients! This section is meant as a general overview of the options and *not* as a treatment guide. *A patient must always see a doctor about appropriate medical treatment.*

Who Should Be Treated for Chronic Hepatitis C?

Not all people with hepatitis C are good candidates for the currently available treatments. The decision to treat or not must be made by a doctor. In most cases, this decision should be made by a specialist familiar with the treatment of chronic hepatitis C or by the patient's primary care doctor in consultation with such a specialist.

Almost all patients with chronic hepatitis C should be *considered* for treatment. *If the diagnosis of chronic hepatitis C is made by a primary care doctor who is not familiar with treatment, the patient should be referred to a specialist.* Although all patients are not necessarily candidates for treatment, most should be evaluated by a specialist experienced with treatment of hepatitis C. Exceptions to this rule include patients with more pressing concurrent illnesses, such as serious heart disease or cancer; elderly patients; and patients with advanced cirrhosis, who should be referred for evaluation for liver transplantation if they are eligible. Many patients with significant depression or mental illness are also poor candidates for treatment, as life-threatening mood alterations and even suicide can occur as a result of receiving currently available treatments. People who are actively abusing illegal drugs or alcohol are generally not good candidates for treatment.

Which patients would liver specialists treat? At present there is no consensus. Some liver specialists will treat virtually all patients with chronic hepatitis C, even those for whom it may be dangerous; others will only treat certain patients. Some liver specialists will not recommend treatment for individuals who have had hepatitis C virus infection for many years and have only minimal inflammation and fibrosis in a liver biopsy. Some think that treatment is not indicated for patients over sixty-five years old, and some published studies support this.

I cannot make specific recommendations about which patients with chronic hepatitis C should be treated. This depends on the judgment of an experienced physician and the individual patient's overall physical and mental health. I can, however, stress a few general points that should be considered, based on what we know about chronic hepatitis C and the currently available drugs.

- Hepatitis C generally progresses very slowly. Those without significant inflammation or fibrosis in their liver biopsies have the option of thinking about treatment, starting at their convenience, and even waiting a few years until newer and more effective drugs may be available.
- Individuals with significant inflammation and fibrosis indicated in their liver biopsies are probably at an increased risk of developing cirrhosis and should probably be treated sooner rather than waiting too long. However, treatment of chronic hepatitis C is *never* an emergency, and a few months' wait will probably not be detrimental to anyone.
- Individuals with cirrhosis evident in their biopsies but no complications should probably consider earlier treatment to prevent progression. However, these patients are a little less likely to respond successfully to currently available treatments or to tolerate them.
- Because hepatitis C is a slowly progressive disease, elderly patients should probably not be treated with currently

available medications. However, "elderly" is tough to define; there is no exact age cutoff. The decision depends on the person's overall state of health and liver biopsy findings.

- People with more pressing physical diseases, mental illness, or social problems that prevent them from complying with a complex treatment regimen should *not* be treated. Some patients with diabetes, thyroid disease, kidney disease, blood disorders, and other conditions may not be able to take interferon alpha.
- Patients with complications of cirrhosis should *not* be treated except perhaps in an approved clinical trial.
- A patient who has received the currently available combination of interferon alpha plus ribavirin, without a successful response, should probably not be treated again with these drugs and should wait until newer drugs are available.

Currently Available Drugs for Chronic Hepatitis C

At present, the Food and Drug Administration (FDA) has approved several different treatments for patients with chronic hepatitis C. Others are likely to be approved soon after or even before this book is published. The approved and soon-to-be-approved drugs and drug combinations are summarized in Table 6.1.

The number of drugs available can be confusing. Much of this confusion results from competition between pharmaceutical companies and government regulatory policies, not for scientific reasons. Three different interferon alphas, produced by three different manufacturers, are approved for chronic hepatitis C. Two peginterferon alphas, produced by two different manufacturers, may be available in the near future. Ribavirin is currently exclusively licensed from one pharmaceutical company to another and only approved for use with one type of interferon alpha. This situation will eventually change, and ribavirin will also likely be approved for use with other interferon alphas. It is available as a "stand-alone" product that doctors can pre-

Table 6.1 FDA-Approved Drugs for Treating Hepatitis C

Generic Name	Trade Name	Manufacturer
Approved		
Interferon alpha-2b	Intron-A	Schering-Plough
Interferon alpha-2b	Roferon	Hoffman La Roche
Interferon alfacon-1	Infergen	Amgen
Interferon alpha-2b/ribavirin combination	Rebetron	Schering-Plough
Peginterferon alpha-2b	Peg-Intron	Schering-Plough
Ribavirin*	Rebetol	Schering-Plough
Likely to Be Approved Soon		
Peginterferon alpha-2a	Pegasys	Hoffman La Roche
Peginterferon alpha-2b/ribavirin combination*	Not yet known	Schering-Plough
Peginterferon alpha-2a/ribavirin combination*	Not yet known	Hoffman La Roche

*At the present time, ribavirin capsules have been approved for use in combination with interferon alpha-2b and peginterferon alpha-2b; however, doctors may prescribe them with any interferon or peginterferon. Ribavirin alone is not effective for the treatment of hepatitis C.

scribe to be used with any available interferon alpha. The choices and combinations of drugs available can be simplified as follows:

1. All interferon alphas, no matter which company manufactures them, work the same. There are no proven, clinically significant differences between interferon alpha-2a, interferon alpha-2b (for you biochemists reading this, the difference is only one conservative amino acid substitution between 2a and 2b), and interferon alfacon-1.
2. Although there are chemical differences between the polyethylene glycol modifications of peginterferon alpha-2a (Pegasys) and peginterferon alpha-2b (Peg-Intron), there are no available data to suggest that peginterferon alpha-2a and peginterferon alpha-2b are different in terms of their safety and efficacy in the treatment of chronic hepatitis C. These two compounds should be considered equivalent unless head-to-head comparisons in clinical trials ever prove otherwise.
3. The active ingredient of peginterferon alpha is still interferon alpha. However, because it is administered less

frequently and gives better blood concentrations of interferon alpha, peginterferon is easier to take and more effective than the unmodified interferon alphas.

4. Ribavirin will work effectively with any interferon alpha.

Interferon Alphas

All approved treatments of chronic hepatitis C depend on the use of interferon alphas. Interferon alphas are proteins naturally produced by the body, especially in response to viral infections. Those currently approved for hepatitis C in the United States are recombinant preparations, produced by using recombinant DNA methodology. They have various effects on the body, including the activation of general antiviral responses and stimulation of the immune system to seek out and kill virus-infected cells. *Interferon alphas were not specifically designed to attack the hepatitis C virus.* They stimulate a wide range of responses and, because of this, have a wide range of side effects.

Interferon alphas were available before the hepatitis C virus was discovered and, in fact, were used in clinical trials to treat patients with non-A, non-B hepatitis. They were selected for use in chronic hepatitis C because of their general antiviral and immune system effects. They were approved for the treatment of chronic hepatitis C because well-designed clinical trials showed that some patients with chronic hepatitis C treated with interferon alpha had decreased liver inflammation. It has also been shown that between 10 and 20 percent of patients treated with interferon alpha for six to eighteen months have no detectable hepatitis C virus in their blood several months after stopping treatment.

Ribavirin

The FDA has also approved the combination of interferon alpha-2b and ribavirin for patients with chronic hepatitis C. Ribavirin is a synthetic compound with activity against several different viruses. *Like interferon alpha, ribavirin was not specifically designed to attack the hepatitis C virus.* Ribavirin had been around for many years before the discovery of the hepatitis C virus and was shown to be effective against several viruses in humans and other animals. In the United States, ribavirin was first approved in aerosol form for the treatment of respiratory syncytial virus, which causes respiratory infections in children. In several studies, oral ribavirin used as a single agent for the treatment of adults with chronic hepatitis C was shown *not* to be effective. However, the combination of interferon alpha and ribavirin was subsequently shown in several studies to be more effective than interferon alpha alone in the treatment of chronic hepatitis C. The combination led to undetectable hepatitis C virus in the blood several months after treatment at a rate of more than twice that of interferon alpha alone (greater than 40 percent compared to less than 20 percent). As a result of these studies, the FDA approved interferon alpha-2b plus ribavirin (Rebetron) for the treatment of chronic hepatitis C.

Peginterferon Alpha

Peginterferon alpha (sometimes referred to as pegylated interferon) is a new preparation of interferon alpha. It is administered by injection. The active ingredient of peginterferon alpha is interferon alpha. It has the same effects as regular interferon alpha against viruses and on the immune system. The difference between peginterferon alpha and unmodified interferon alpha is in its pharmacokinetics (absorption and elimination from the body) and not its pharmacodynamics (mechanism of action). By attaching a polyethylene glycol molecule to the interferon molecule, it is eliminated more slowly from the body. As a result, the drug can be administered less frequently (generally one injection a week compared to three injections a week for unmodified interferon alpha) and more constant and effective concentrations are achieved in the blood (see Figure 6.1). Less frequent injections generally lead to better patient compliance. More constant effective blood concentrations may also lead to greater antiviral efficacy.

What Drugs to Use?

Keeping it as simple as possible, what treatment should a patient try? Preliminary data suggest that the response rates are better with

Figure 6.1 Differences in Interferon Alpha Blood Levels

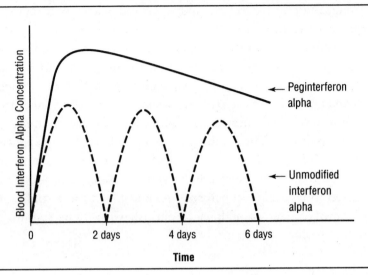

ribavirin and a peginterferon compared to an unmodified interferon and ribavirin. The once-a-week dosing of peginterferon is also better for most patients. *A peginterferon alpha and ribavirin will probably be the first treatment of choice for most patients with chronic hepatitis C until superior drugs are available.*

Some individuals cannot take ribavirin. These are patients with anemia, kidney failure, and heart disease. Ribavirin can cause modest to serious anemia. Patients with significant heart disease could be at risk for a heart attack if they become suddenly anemic as a result of taking ribavirin. For this reason, people with known heart disease or risk factors for it should have a cardiac stress test before taking the drug. Since the kidneys excrete ribavirin, it should not be used in individuals with significant kidney disease, except perhaps in approved clinical trials. For patients who cannot take ribavirin, treatment with a peginterferon alpha alone is currently the next best choice.

Administration of Currently Available Drugs

Alpha interferons either come as powders that must be mixed with sterile water before use or as premixed solutions. They are stable if stored in the refrigerator. Interferon alpha, unmodified or pegylated, is administered by subcutaneous (under the skin) or intramuscular (into the muscle) injections. Most patients administer the injections themselves, with small syringes and needles similar to those used by diabetics to inject insulin or with an injection pen supplied with the drug. Most people choose to inject the interferon into their thighs; however, other areas such as the abdomen can work. Patients should obtain training from a doctor or nurse before injecting themselves.

Peginterferon alpha is generally injected once a week. Unmodified interferons are generally injected every other day, three times a week. *The doses of the different unmodified and peginterferon alphas vary depending on the different manufacturers' preparations; a patient must follow his or her doctor's instructions carefully.* For unmodified interferon alpha, the single dose is three million units (units are a measurement of the drug's activity) or the equivalent of three million units in micrograms. Peginterferons are dosed on a mass basis in micrograms, and the amounts vary for the different preparations. One manufacturer recommends weight-based dosing, in which the amount of peginterferon injected each week depends on the patient's weight. Again, patients injecting interferon, unmodified or pegylated, should pay careful attention to their doctors' instructions regarding appropriate doses.

Ribavirin for chronic hepatitis C comes as 200-milligram (0.2-gram) capsules. The capsules are stable at room temperature. Ribavirin is taken two times every day, in the morning and at night. The recommended dose is usually two capsules in the morning and three in the evening (total 1 gram) for individuals who weigh less than 165 pounds (75 kilograms) and three tablets in the morning and three in the evening (1.2 grams) for individuals who weigh 165 pounds (75 kilograms) or more.

Interferon alpha-based treatments for chronic hepatitis C are generally given for six to twelve months. Some doctors will treat individuals infected with genotypes other than type 1 for six months and those with genotype 1 for twelve months. The ideal duration of treatment is still not entirely clear, but few doctors will administer the drugs for more than one year.

Before treatment with interferon, with or without ribavirin, patients should have a battery of blood tests to make sure that there are no contraindications to receiving the drugs. If thyroid disease, diabetes mellitus, or kidney disease are suspected based on blood testing, treatment should be deferred until these conditions are investigated further. Anemia, a low white blood count, and a low platelet count may also make a patient ineligible for treatment with interferon alpha or ribavirin.

Goals of Treatment

Before explaining the goals of treatment, I must define some of the jargon that has caught on regarding the therapy of chronic hepatitis C. These terms are not all scientifically accurate or precise, and they are sometimes confusing. Nonetheless, most doctors and many patients use them.

The first thing that needs to be clarified is the parameter that is measured to gauge a response to treatment (see Table 6.2). The most commonly used parameter of response to treatment is loss of hepatitis C virus RNA from the blood when measured by polymerase chain reaction (PCR) testing, or *virological response*. In earlier studies, before routine RNA testing was readily available, response to treatment was defined as normalization of blood ALT activities, called a *biochemical response*. Measuring blood ALT activity is not an ideal way to determine response to treatment because in some patients it may be elevated for reasons other than hepatitis C, such as excessive alcohol consumption or fatty liver. Another type of response that is sometimes measured in studies but rarely in the routine care of patients is called a *histological response*. This is determined by decreased inflammation and possibly fibrosis seen in a liver biopsy

Table 6.2 Responses to Treatment for Chronic Hepatitis C

Term	Definition
Virological response	Undetectable hepatitis C viral RNA in blood by PCR
Biochemical response	Normalization of blood ALT activity
Histological response	Improvement in inflammation and possibly fibrosis in a liver biopsy

after treatment. In routine clinical practice today, a sustained virological response is generally regarded as the desired goal of treatment.

Additional terminology is used to define the nature of the measured response (see Table 6.3). The goal of treatment is to become a *sustained responder*. Sustained responders have undetectable hepatitis C virus RNA in the blood six months and longer after stopping treatment. It is presumed, although not yet strictly proven, that many such individuals will have cleared the virus from their bodies and that the liver inflammation from hepatitis C will stop. This may not be strictly true as the hepatitis C virus may be present in the liver at very low levels after treatment; the virus is just not replicating rapidly enough to produce significant levels in the blood. It is also possible that an apparent sustained response may be transient and that hepatitis C virus RNA will again become detectable in blood more than six months after stopping treatment. For this reason, sustained responders should probably have PCR testing for virus in their blood performed every year or so for at least a few years after treatment is stopped.

Many, perhaps most, patients with chronic hepatitis C treated with an interferon alpha-based therapy have a virological response

Table 6.3 Responses to Treatment for Hepatitis C

These terms are generally used to describe a specific virological response.

Term	Definition
Responder	A patient who has undetectable viral RNA in blood
Nonresponder	A patient who has detectable viral RNA in blood during treatment
Relapser	A patient who responded to treatment and then had detectable serum virus RNA after treatment was discontinued
Treatment failure	Nonresponder or relapser
Sustained responder	A patient with undetectable viral RNA in blood six months and longer after stopping treatment
Partial responder	A patient whose blood viral RNA concentration decreases significantly during treatment but in whom it is still detectable; or a patient who has a normalization of blood ALT during treatment but still has detectable viral RNA
Breakthrough	A patient who is an initial responder to treatment, then develops detectable viral RNA in blood later during the course of treatment

during treatment, and then relapse after treatment is stopped. *Relapsers* are patients who have undetectable hepatitis C virus RNA in their blood during treatment that becomes detectable after stopping the drugs. The long-term consequences of having a response during treatment and then relapsing are not clear. Some studies suggest that these patients may have decreased inflammation, according to liver biopsies obtained after treatment. The significance of this in terms of a long-term prognosis is not clear.

Roughly a third of patients treated with interferon alpha-based therapy will be *nonresponders*. In nonresponders, hepatitis C viral RNA will persist in the blood during treatment. Some of the initial responders will experience a *breakthrough* during treatment, and viral RNA will be detected in the blood later during the course of therapy. Some will be considered *partial responders* because their blood hepatitis C viral RNA concentrations will decrease but not become undetectable by PCR testing. Most liver specialists generally group partial responders and individuals who break through with nonresponders, because they never had persistently undetectable hepatitis C viral RNA in the blood during treatment.

Although a sustained virological response is the goal of most doctors and patients, it is possible that treatment with interferon alpha, with or without ribavirin, *may* be beneficial even if this goal is not attained. Some studies suggest that treatment slows the development of fibrosis. Others suggest that interferon alpha may prevent the development of hepatocellular carcinoma in patients with hepatitis C and cirrhosis. However, longer term studies are necessary to confirm the benefits of treatment in those who are not sustained responders.

Although it seems obvious that achieving a sustained virological response is of benefit to a patient, rigorous, long-term studies still must be completed to definitively prove this. Very preliminary case reports of just a few patients with chronic hepatitis C examined ten or more years after achieving a sustained response to interferon alpha have shown that none have developed cirrhosis. However, formal, long-term studies of such patients, with relevant comparison groups, remain to be completed. In the meantime, I believe that patients can assume that a sustained virological response to treatment predicts a long-term benefit in most instances.

First-Time Treatment of Chronic Hepatitis C

Patients with chronic hepatitis C who have never been treated previously are called *naive*. Today, most naive patients who have chronic hepatitis C and are good candidates for treatment should receive a combination of interferon alpha and ribavirin. Most doctors will use peginterferon alpha with ribavirin. Those patients who for some reason cannot tolerate ribavirin should probably be treated with peginterferon alpha alone.

How do naive patients with chronic hepatitis C respond to treatment? About two thirds of patients will be responders to treatment, meaning that blood hepatitis C virus RNA will not be detectable during treatment. This value is probably about the same for patients receiving unmodified interferon alpha alone, peginterferon alpha alone, or an unmodified or peginterferon plus ribavirin.

At the completion of treatment, blood testing should be performed to measure hepatitis C viral RNA by PCR. Patients without detectable viral RNA by PCR testing at the completion of treatment are called *end-of-treatment responders*. In these patients, PCR testing for viral RNA should be performed again six months after stopping therapy. Patients who do not have detectable blood viral RNA six months after finishing treatment are called sustained responders, or *long-term responders*. But these patients may relapse and again have detectable viral RNA in the blood. Therefore, blood RNA concentrations should probably be checked periodically, perhaps every six to twelve months for a few years after treatment is stopped.

How many patients will be sustained responders and have no detectable serum hepatitis C virus RNA in the blood six months or longer after treatment? In patients treated with an unmodified interferon alpha alone for six months, the answer is less than 20 percent. Treatment for a year with unmodified interferon alpha improves the sustained response rate to almost 20 percent. In patients treated with interferon alpha-2b plus ribavirin for six to twelve months, the sustained response rate is approximately 40 to 47 percent. Preliminary studies show that the sustained response rates with a peginterferon alpha plus ribavirin for one year is approximately 50 percent, or slightly greater. These results, some of which come from unpublished preliminary data, are summarized in Table 6.4.

Table 6.4 Sustained Response Rates to Treatment Regimens

Treatment Regimen	Sustained Response Rate
Interferon alpha (6 months)	Less than 20%
Interferon alpha ($\geq$ 12 months)	Approaching 20%
Peginterferon alpha (12 months)	Approximately 30%
Interferon alpha plus ribavirin (12 months)	Approximately 40%
Peginterferon alpha plus ribavirin (12 months)	Approximately 50%

There are several predictors for which patients with chronic hepatitis C are more likely to respond to treatment. In general, the following are correlated with a *lower* probability of responding: age greater than forty-five years, duration of infection longer than five years, the presence of fibrosis or cirrhosis in a liver biopsy, infection with genotypes 1a or 1b, and higher blood hepatitis C virus RNA concentrations (viral loads) at the start of treatment. Despite these facts, it is not possible to apply these predictors to an individual patient to calculate his or her exact chance of responding to treatment. A doctor may be able to better guess ahead of time who is more or less likely to respond but cannot make such predictions with certainty in an individual patient.

In summary, individuals with chronic hepatitis C who are good candidates for currently available treatments have about a 50 percent overall chance of achieving a sustained response of no detectable viral RNA in the blood after treatment with peginterferon plus ribavirin. For those infected with non–type 1 genotypes, it is slightly higher. A fifty-fifty chance isn't that bad, but better treatments are clearly needed.

Retreatment

One of the big issues in the treatment of patients with chronic hepatitis C is what to offer patients who are nonresponders or relapsers after a first course of treatment. The current options are basically limited to:

1. Retreatment with interferon alpha and ribavirin or peginterferon alpha and ribavirin for patients who received interferon alpha alone for their first course of treatment.
2. Retreatment with interferon alpha, at a higher dose and/or for a longer duration, with or without ribavirin.
3. Enrollment in approved clinical trials of different interferon-based treatment protocols.

Retreatment of Relapsers Who Received Interferon Alpha Alone

The results of clinical trials clearly show that the combination of interferon alpha plus ribavirin improves the response rate of relapsers who were previously treated with interferon alpha alone. In the first published study of 345 patients who were relapsers after treatment with interferon alpha alone, 45.7 percent who were retreated with interferon alpha plus ribavirin had a sustained response of undetectable blood hepatitis C virus RNA six months after stopping therapy. The results are likely to be the same or perhaps slightly better for peginterferon plus ribavirin. For patients with chronic hepatitis C who relapse after treatment with interferon alone, retreatment with the combination of interferon alpha plus ribavirin is a good option. The treatment of relapsers to interferon alpha alone was in fact the first indication for which combination therapy with interferon alpha-2b plus ribavirin was approved by the FDA.

Retreatment of Nonresponders Who Received Interferon Alpha Alone

Retreatment of nonresponders to interferon alpha alone remains problematic. Many liver specialists will offer retreatment with interferon alpha or peginterferon alpha plus ribavirin to nonresponders. Overall, the retreatment rate of such subjects is quite low, somewhere between 5 and 15 percent. However, the results with interferon plus ribavirin for nonresponders infected with genotypes other than type 1 appear to reflect a higher percent. On the other hand, the results for those infected with genotype 1 are probably around 5 percent. Therefore, it may be reasonable for nonresponders to interferon alpha alone to be retreated with interferon alpha or peginterferon alpha plus ribavirin if they are infected with hepatitis C viral genotypes other than type 1.

Many other variations of available drugs have been studied for the retreatment of nonresponders to interferon alpha. These studies have examined virtually every combination imaginable of interferon alpha, peginterferon alpha, and ribavirin at various doses and for various durations. Except for a few isolated studies, the overall results have not been very promising.

In summary, treatment of nonresponders to interferon alpha is difficult. Some data suggest that those infected with non–type 1 genotypes will benefit from a second course of treatment with interferon alpha or peginterferon alpha plus ribavirin. Otherwise, the best options may be for such patients to wait a few years for hopefully better treatments or to enroll in a clinical trial (see Chapter 9).

Relapsers and Nonresponders to Interferon Alpha Plus Ribavirin

What about patients with chronic hepatitis C who have failed to respond to treatment with interferon alpha (unmodified or pegylated) with ribavirin? At present, no specific recommendations can be made. Such patients may want to consider participating in clinical trials; however, most right now only involve various types of interferon and ribavirin. In most cases, the most reasonable option is probably observation until new and more promising drugs are available. The choice among these options depends on the particular patient and his or her doctor. Regardless of the choice, patients should realize that most people with chronic hepatitis C do well in the long term, with or without treatment.

Side Effects of Treatment

There are numerous side effects associated with all the preparations of interferon alpha. For this reason, careful monitoring is necessary during treatment. Because low blood counts are a potential side effect, patients should have their blood drawn and complete blood counts and platelet counts checked one, two, and four weeks after treatment is started and roughly once a month thereafter. Blood ALT activity, bilirubin concentration, and albumin concentration should also be checked periodically during therapy. Patients should see their doctors or a nurse at least once every few months during treatment and contact their doctors if they experience side effects.

Common and potentially serious side effects of interferon alpha at the doses generally used to treat patients with chronic hepatitis C are low neutrophil counts and low platelet counts. Neutrophils, also called granulocytes, are a particular type of white blood cell important in fighting bacterial infections. Platelets, which are involved in blood clotting, may also be low in individuals with cirrhosis. As mentioned, patients should have their blood counts monitored during treatment with interferon alpha. If the neutrophil count falls below 750 cells per cubic millimeter of blood, or the platelet count falls below 50,000 cells per cubic millimeter of blood, the daily dose can be reduced until these values rise above these levels. If the neutrophil count falls below 500 cells per cubic millimeter of blood or the platelet count falls below 30,000 cells per cubic millimeter of blood, interferon therapy should probably be discontinued. Resumption of treatment can be considered when the blood counts return to their baseline values.

There are many other side effects of interferon alpha therapy besides low blood counts. The most common is the development of flulike symptoms. These can be quite severe and include fever, cold sweats, shaking chills, muscle aches and pains, and joint aches and pains. Flulike symptoms are usually worse near the start of treatment and less common later in the course of therapy. To help tolerate mild to moderate flulike symptoms, I generally recommend that patients inject the interferon about an hour before going to sleep and take acetaminophen (Tylenol) right before injecting the interferon. The acetaminophen will provide some relief of the symptoms and, if taken at bedtime, possibly help the patient sleep through the night. Flulike symptoms rarely require stopping treatment, but on occasion they are so intolerable that there is no other option but to stop.

Interferon alpha treatment can aggravate diabetes mellitus and thyroid disorders. Patients with diabetes mellitus who are treated with interferon alpha should carefully monitor their blood sugars. Patients with thyroid disease (and possibly all treated patients) should have blood tests of thyroid function checked periodically during treatment. Significant abnormalities in blood sugar or thyroid tests may necessitate stopping treatment. Patients with preexisting thyroid disease and poorly controlled diabetes may not be able to tolerate interferon alpha.

Psychiatric problems, some severe, have been reported in individuals being treated for hepatitis C. Severe depression, including suicide, has occurred in patients with chronic hepatitis C treated with interferon alpha with or without ribavirin. Patients with serious preexisting depression or other psychiatric disorders probably should not be treated with interferon alpha. Those with a history of depression or other psychiatric illnesses should probably be evaluated by a psychiatrist before treatment is initiated and during treatment if it is started. If severe depression develops during treatment, the drugs should be immediately discontinued and the patient closely followed and referred to a psychiatrist as necessary. If more mild signs of depression occur, the addition of an antidepressant medication during treatment may be helpful. The main thing to remember is that depression can be very serious, even life threatening. If depression becomes severe during treatment, the best response is always to stop the interferon plus ribavirin, as the treatment of chronic hepatitis C is never an emergency.

Irritability, confusion, nervousness, impaired concentration, anxiety, and insomnia may all occur in individuals taking interferon alpha and may occur more commonly when interferon is combined with ribavirin. Sometimes these psychiatric problems are so severe that treatment must be stopped. As with depression, psychiatric consultation should be considered if these symptoms become significant. If in doubt about the severity of the psychiatric symptoms, the drugs should be stopped.

Virtually every other complaint imaginable has been reported by patients receiving interferon alpha with or without ribavirin. Some of the more frequent side effects, which are usually not severe, include fever, rashes, headache, muscle aches, fatigue, back pain, dry mouth, nausea, diarrhea, tingling in the arms and legs, temporary hair loss, and inflammation at the injection site. These usually are mild to moderate and do not require stopping treatment. Occasionally, patients have an apparent allergic reaction to interferon alpha, and the drug must be discontinued if this occurs. Despite the numerous side effects, interferon alpha therapy is generally safe if patients are followed closely by their doctors. Most patients complete the prescribed course of therapy.

The major side effect caused by ribavirin is the rapid development of *hemolytic anemia*. This is a sudden drop in the red blood cell count, hemoglobin, and hematocrit that results from the rupture of red blood cells. For this reason, the blood count must be monitored one, two, and four weeks after starting therapy and monthly thereafter. If the hemoglobin concentration drops below 10 milligrams per deciliter during treatment, the dose of ribavirin should be cut in half until it returns to normal. If the hemoglobin concentration drops below 8.5 milligrams per deciliter, ribavirin treatment should be discontinued. Because sudden-onset anemia can be very dangerous in individuals with heart disease, patients known to have significant heart disease should not receive ribavirin. Patients at risk for heart disease should be evaluated with a stress test prior to treatment.

Ribavirin may cause birth defects. Pregnant women should not take ribavirin. Men who are taking ribavirin should not impregnate their female sexual partners.

Things to Remember About Current Treatment of Chronic Hepatitis C

The primary goal of treatment for patients with chronic hepatitis C is to eradicate the virus from the body. This is only achieved in about half of all patients. Most data from published studies are only available for six months after treatment and sustained response rates *may* be lower with longer term follow-up. If the virus is eradicated from the body, the progression of liver disease will very likely stop.

The secondary goal of treatment is to slow the progression of liver disease, even if a sustained virological response is not achieved. This is less easy to assess. Even if the virus is not eradicated from the body, transient improvements in liver inflammation and possibly even fibrosis are sometimes obtained. Although long-term follow-up is not available, partially successful treatment *may* slow or halt the progression to cirrhosis. Some studies have also suggested that treatment of patients with cirrhosis caused by hepatitis C *may* have a lower incidence in the development of hepatocellular carcinoma after several years of follow-up.

Patients and their doctors must realize that the treatment of chronic hepatitis C is rapidly evolving and subject to radical change. Many clinical studies are still in progress to optimize available interferon-based treatments. Most important, many pharmaceutical companies, biotechnology companies, and academic laboratories are working on novel drugs to attack the hepatitis C virus and prevent the complications resulting from infection (see Chapter 9). When such drugs are developed, they will add greater specificity to the treatment of hepatitis C and will either complement, or hopefully be used instead of, the currently available interferon alpha-based therapies. It is unlikely that these novel drugs, which for the most part are still in the laboratory, will be available in the immediate future. Like all new drugs, they must first be tested in approved clinical trials to prove their safety and efficacy.

The important take-home messages about the treatment of chronic hepatitis C for patients and their doctors are:

1. Treatment of chronic hepatitis C is never an emergency. Chronic hepatitis C is a slowly progressive disease and does not progress to cirrhosis in most patients. There is always time to think about treatment, whether and when to start it, and if it is the right choice.
2. Treatment can always be stopped once started if problems or significant side effects occur.
3. Treatment of patients with chronic hepatitis C with interferon alpha or interferon alpha plus ribavirin is imperfect and only about half of all patients achieve the desired sustained response.

4. Different doctors will recommend different durations of treatment with different preparations of interferon alpha, peginterferon alpha, and ribavirin. There is no single approach agreed upon by all doctors. A particular doctor's judgment and biases, and the patient's wishes, are important factors in determining the exact treatment plan.
5. The current trend favored by most doctors for the treatment of chronic hepatitis C is peginterferon alpha plus ribavirin. The addition of ribavirin to interferon alpha clearly improves sustained response rate compared to interferon alpha alone.
6. Patients who relapse after a first course of interferon alpha alone should be considered for retreatment with interferon alpha plus ribavirin. The retreatment options for non-responders to interferon alpha, or for relapsers and non-responders to interferon alpha plus ribavirin are less clear. The best choices for such patients may be to wait for new drugs. They may enroll in clinical trials, but most trials still rely primarily on the use of interferon alpha.
7. Although a sustained virological response (eradication of the virus from the body) is a major goal of therapy, treatment may be associated with other benefits such as a decrease in the chance of developing cirrhosis or hepatocellular carcinoma.
8. Patients who do not respond to presently available treatments should remain optimistic. New drugs will likely be available in the next few years (see Chapter 9).

Treatment of Special Groups of Patients

Certain groups of patients with chronic hepatitis C require special consideration when discussing treatment. These groups include active substance abusers and those concurrently infected with other viruses such as the hepatitis B virus and HIV. *The patient with chronic hepatitis C who already has complications of cirrhosis usually needs to focus on the potentially serious problems caused by the failing liver rather than treatment of the underlying hepatitis C.*

The Alcohol and Drug Abuser with Chronic Hepatitis C

Current treatment protocols for chronic hepatitis C require good compliance, frequent medical monitoring, and the injection of medications. It is almost impossible to treat an active alcohol or drug abuser for chronic hepatitis C. *In nearly all such cases, the substance abuse should be treated first.*

The cornerstone of treatment of the individual with alcohol abuse is *complete and unconditional abstinence from alcohol.* The same is true for any substance abuse disorder. *No medication or procedure is a substitute for abstinence.* However, abstinence from alcohol or another drug is often easier said than done. Substance abuse and dependence are diseases, and a major component of these diseases is an inability to stop using the substance despite knowing that it is harmful. For individuals with alcohol and other substance dependence problems, hospital admission for detoxification may be required. In many cases, detoxification should ideally be followed up with inpatient rehabilitation, usually for at least one month. Additional outpatient psychotherapy or participation in day programs is often necessary for some patients. For alcohol abusers, participation in Alcoholics Anonymous should probably be continued for life. Other substance abusers may benefit from Narcotics Anonymous, a similar type program. Despite these actions, the relapse rates for alcohol and drug abusers are quite high.

Remember, the treatment of chronic hepatitis C is never an emergency. Administration of the available treatment to active drug or alcohol abusers is difficult and poses risks. Treatment requires patients to pay careful attention to instructions and to have regular medical follow-ups, which active substance abusers may have trouble doing. Drug abusers may forget that they have taken their medication and mistakenly double their dose, causing numerous side effects. The underlying substance abuse disorders must be treated first and the patient must be off drugs or alcohol for a reasonable period of time, probably at least six months, before treatment is initiated.

Hepatitis C Virus and Human Immunodeficiency Virus (HIV) Infection

So-called coinfection with hepatitis C virus and HIV is not unusual. Many years ago, chronic hepatitis C was not treated in individuals infected with HIV, as their life expectancy was short. However, since the recent revolution in the treatment of HIV with nucleoside analogues and protease inhibitors, patients have been living long and productive lives. Some have been living long enough to develop complications of cirrhosis from hepatitis C.

In general, patients with HIV infection and a healthy immune system (normal CD4 or "T-cell" counts) and no complications from AIDS, who also have chronic hepatitis C, should probably be approached just like a patient with chronic hepatitis C without HIV infection. Equally aggressive diagnostic procedures and treatments should be considered in patients with hepatitis C virus and HIV co-infection without laboratory evidence of a compromised immune system or AIDS. However, since such patients take numerous different drugs, there is the potential for drug interactions and compliance problems. Patients on several drugs to treat HIV and two drugs to treat hepatitis C are at an increased risk for developing side effects and should be monitored closely.

In individuals with very low CD4 counts or with AIDS, a less aggressive approach to hepatitis C is usually indicated. In such patients, other problems may be more immediate. The approach to each patient depends on that particular case and the doctor's judgment. More aggresive treatment of chronic hepatitis C could be considered if an individual with AIDS becomes stable on anti-HIV medications.

Hepatitis C Virus and Hepatitis B Virus Infection

The hepatitis B virus and hepatitis C virus are transmitted in similar fashions. In Western countries, hepatitis B virus infection is less common than hepatitis C. In Eastern countries and parts of Africa, the opposite is true. In patients with both, the two diseases should be approached together. Many of the diagnostic and treatment considerations are similar. Patients should probably first be treated for hepatitis B, then for hepatitis C (for more information on hepatitis B, see *The Liver Disorders Sourcebook*). However, the order of treatment, and whether treatment of both viruses can be attempted together with different drugs, is not entirely clear. People eligible for treatment for both hepatitis B and hepatitis C should see a specialist who has experience in treating both conditions.

The Patient with Cirrhosis and Complications

Individuals with chronic hepatitis C and early cirrhosis detectable only in a liver biopsy should be considered for treatment just like patients without cirrhosis. However, patients with more advanced cases of cirrhosis from hepatitis C are another matter. Treatment of the underlying hepatitis C in such patients is often not possible and should probably not be considered. If it is, such patients should only be treated in approved clinical trials. In patients with complications of cirrhosis, the risks of treating chronic hepatitis C with interferon alpha, with or without ribavirin, generally outweigh the benefits. Patients with complications of cirrhosis are much more likely to suffer serious adverse events during treatment. And these patients already suffer precisely from what treatment aims to prevent in the long term: the complications of cirrhosis.

Patients with complications of cirrhosis need to be treated for those complications (see Table 6.5). When cirrhosis is advanced, some of the complications become nearly impossible to treat or prevent. This condition is commonly referred to as end-stage liver disease. In end-stage liver disease, liver transplantation is the only option. Hence, periodic careful follow-up by a doctor knowledgeable in liver diseases is important. If the complications of cirrhosis become uncontrollable, or when an experienced physician realizes that they will soon become so, referral to a liver transplantation center is essential. Fortunately, in many cases, the complications of cirrhosis respond to the various interventions described below.

Table 6.5 Treatments for Complications of Cirrhosis

Complication	Treatment
Bleeding from esophageal varices	Endoscopic sclerotherapy
	Endoscopic rubber band ligation
	Beta-blockers and possibly nitrates
	Vasopressin and somatostatin analogue (emergencies only)
	Balloon compression (emergencies only)
	Transjugular intrahepatic portosystemic shunt (TIPS)
	Surgical portal-systemic shunts
Edema and ascites	Low-sodium diet (very important)
	Diuretics (spironolactone usually first choice)
	Paracentesis (removal of ascites with needle)
Encephalopathy	Low-protein diet
	Lactulose
	Neomycin
Bleeding tendencies	Vitamin K
	Fresh frozen plasma (emergencies or prior to some procedures)
Spontaneous bacterial peritonitis	Antibiotics
Hyponatremia (low blood sodium concentration)	Restriction of water intake

Bleeding from Esophageal or Gastric Varices

Bleeding from esophageal or gastric varices (varicose veins of the esophagus or stomach) is a life-threatening emergency that must be treated immediately. Intravenous fluid and blood must be given promptly if the patient is not stable. The diagnosis is generally made by *endoscopy*. In endoscopy, a fiber-optic tube is inserted into the patient's esophagus, then passed into the stomach and first part of the small intestine. This gives the doctor a direct view of the bleeding varices and other possible sources of bleeding.

If bleeding esophageal varices are identified during the endoscopic examination, sclerotherapy or rubber band ligation are usually the first-line treatments. Both of these procedures are done through the endoscope. Sclerotherapy is accomplished by injection of a caustic substance into the varicose vein. In rubber band ligation, rubber bands are tied (ligated) around varices to stop bleeding and obliterate them. Gastric varices cannot be treated by sclerotherapy because the caustic chemical can irritate the stomach and cause it to rupture. Gastric varices can sometimes be treated by rubber band ligation.

Sclerotherapy or rubber band ligation should only be done on patients who have varices that are actively bleeding or have bled previously. If varices are detected incidentally but they have never bled, these treatments are not indicated. If sclerotherapy or rubber band ligation stops variceal bleeding, follow-up endoscopy should be performed on a regular schedule and repeat courses of sclerotherapy or rubber band ligation should be performed until all visible esophageal varices are obliterated.

Beta-blockers and nitrates are oral drugs used to prevent bleeding from esophageal and gastric varices. Several studies have shown that these medications can decrease the incidence of bleeding or rebleeding from esophageal varices. Once the acute bleeding is stopped, or if varices that have not yet bled are found on an endoscopic examination, beta-blockers and sometimes nitrates should be prescribed for the patient.

Endoscopic sclerotherapy or rubber band ligation cannot always stop acute bleeding from esophageal or gastric varices. In some cases, bleeding may be from a condition known as *portal gastropathy* in which the pressure is increased diffusely in the veins of the stomach but there is no single prominent varicose vein to ligate. In these cases, the patient should be admitted to an intensive care unit where medical therapy with vasopressin or somatostatin may be attempted. These medications constrict some blood vessels and/or lower portal pressures.

If acute bleeding from esophageal varices does not stop despite attempted endoscopic and medical treatment, balloon compression may be used as a lifesaving option. A tube with a large balloon at the end is inserted into the esophagus and the balloon is then inflated. The inflated balloon may stop bleeding by direct compression.

Shunts are surgical connections that are made between the portal circulation, which has increased pressure in cirrhosis, and the systemic circulation. Shunts can stop bleeding from gastric or esophageal varices in individuals with cirrhosis and portal hypertension because they lower the blood pressure in the portal system. In classic open surgical shunt procedures, a major vein of the portal circulation is directly connected to a major vein of the lower-pressure systemic circulation. For example, the portal vein may be connected directly to the vena cava, or the splenic vein, which is connected via the portal vein, to a vein leading to a kidney. Such connections allow some portal blood to bypass the cirrhotic liver and lower the pressure in the portal system. This decompresses the esophageal and gastric varices, making them much less likely to bleed. The major complication of surgical shunts is worsening of hepatic encephalopathy, as a larger portion of blood from the gut bypasses the liver and cannot be detoxified.

Today, surgical shunt procedures are rarely performed. More recently, a less invasive shunt procedure has been developed and is generally performed by radiologists. This procedure is known as *transjugular intrahepatic portosystemic shunt*, or TIPS. In TIPS, a hollow tube is placed directly into the liver from an approach through the jugular vein in the neck. The tube is situated to directly connect the portal vein and hepatic vein through the liver, allowing some of the blood to bypass the cirrhotic architecture and relieve pressure in the portal circulation. Patients undergoing TIPS are also at increased risk for developing worsening hepatic encephalopathy after the procedure. In addition, the shunt may clot with time, again increasing the risk of bleeding from gastric or esophageal varices. Despite these complications, TIPS can be life saving.

Edema and Ascites

Edema is retention of fluid in the body. *Ascites* is edema in the abdominal cavity. *The most important, initial therapeutic intervention to prevent ascites and edema in cirrhosis is a strict, low-salt diet.* In individuals with significant ascites and edema, a daily allowance of 500 to 1,000 milligrams of sodium chloride (salt) is ideal, however, most patients find such a diet terribly unpalatable.

Nonetheless, it is important that the patient do everything possible to significantly restrict salt consumption. Virtually all canned and processed foods should be avoided. Meat and fish should only be consumed in small quantities as these foods contain significant quantities of salt. A patient with cirrhosis and ascites should generally stick to a mostly vegetarian diet with low-salt fruits, grains, pastas, and vegetables providing most of the calories. An occasional egg and infrequent small portions of meat may be consumed, but *no* cured or processed meats, such as salami or pastrami. The bottom line is that the patient should eat as salt-free a diet as possible and reduce the intake of foods, including meats, that have a high salt content. If a cirrhotic patient with ascites and edema also has *hyponatremia* (low blood sodium concentration), intake of water should also be restricted, usually to one quart a day or less until the blood sodium concentration returns to near normal.

If diet alone does not control edema and ascites, the next step is to add a diuretic. Diuretics should *not* be used as a substitute for a low-salt diet but are complementary measures. The first-choice diuretic is usually spironolactone (Aldactone). Spironolactone works by counteracting the effects of aldosterone, a hormone that acts on the kidney where blood levels are abnormally increased (in cirrhotic individuals with ascites and edema). If spironolactone and diet do not control ascites and edema, a second diuretic medication, either hydrocholrothiazide or a so-called loop diuretic, such as furosemide (Lasix), is added next. Patients with cirrhosis who are taking diuretics should be followed closely by their doctors to watch for excessive intravascular dehydration, and their kidney function and electrolytes should be periodically checked.

If diet and diuretics do not relieve ascites and the abdominal swelling becomes so intense that it is painful, or if the patient has difficulty breathing from compression on the diaphragm, large-volume *paracentesis* is an option. In this procedure, a needle is inserted into the abdomen through the skin and the fluid is gradually drained. About 4 to 6 liters (1 liter is roughly 1 quart) can be drained at a time. Sometimes, an infusion of albumin will be given at the time the paracentesis is performed. In some patients with advanced cirrhosis, repeated large-volume paracenteses are required.

A type of surgical procedure is available in refractory ascites that cannot be managed by recurrent, large-volume paracentesis treatments. This procedure is associated with serious complications and is very rarely used. The surgical procedure, known as a Denver or a Laveen shunt, places a tube with a one-way valve between the intra-abdominal space and a large vein. As a result, the ascites fluid drains directly into the patient's bloodstream. Serious complications such as infection, clotting of the shunt, and disseminated intravascular coagulation (abnormal clotting of the blood within the circulation) are common after this procedure. Denver or Laveen shunts are usually reserved as last-resort comfort measures for individuals who have massive ascites and who are not eligible for liver transplantation.

Spontaneous Bacterial Peritonitis

Patients with ascites are at risk for *spontaneous bacterial peritonitis* (SBP), an infection of the ascites with bacteria. This infection should be considered in any patient with ascites who develops fever or abdominal pain. Sometimes, spontaneous bacterial peritonitis will present as a general deterioration in overall condition or worsening hepatic encephalopathy in the absence of fever. The diagnostic procedure for spontaneous bacterial peritonitis is paracentesis. Usually, only a small volume of ascites fluid needs to be removed with a needle and syringe. The diagnosis of spontaneous bacterial peritonitis is made if the white blood cell count in the ascites fluid is elevated. Treatment with antibiotics is essential, usually by the intravenous route in the hospital. Some studies have suggested that long-term oral antibiotics may be useful to prevent subsequent infections in individuals with recurrent episodes of spontaneous bacterial peritonitis.

Hepatic Encephalopathy

Hepatic encephalopathy refers to the mental changes that occur as the liver fails. They can range from mild confusion to deep coma. The first step in the treatment of hepatic encephalopathy is a low-protein diet. Proteins are high in nitrogen content. Ammonia and other nitrogen-containing compounds, which are toxic to the brain when not removed by the cirrhotic liver, are produced by the metabolism of proteins by bacteria in the colon. Meats, nuts, and other high-protein foods should be consumed only in very low quantities. Substitute vegetables, fruits, grains, and pastas. This diet is similar to the low-salt diet for ascites and edema.

The first-line drug treatment for hepatic encephalopathy is usually lactulose. Lactulose is a sugar that is not absorbed from the gut. In part, it acts as a laxative helping to expel nitrogen-containing compounds from the colon before bacteria can metabolize them into substances that can be toxic to an individual with a liver that cannot adequately clear them from the blood. Lactulose also makes the inside of the gut more acid, making it less favorable for nitrogen-containing toxins and ammonia to be absorbed. Another drug treatment for encephalopathy is neomycin, an antibiotic that is not absorbed from the gut and kills bacteria in the colon that produce ammonia and other potentially toxic nitrogen-containing compounds.

Bleeding Tendencies

Administration of vitamin K can sometimes help with the decreased production of clotting factors in patients with advanced cirrhosis. In emergency bleeding situations, or prior to invasive medical procedures that may be necessary, fresh frozen plasma can be transfused intravenously. Plasma, the component of blood from which the red and white cells have been removed, contains clotting factors and other proteins. Platelet transfusions may also be given to patients with very low platelet counts to help stop or prevent bleeding.

Liver Transplantation

In some patients, the complications of cirrhosis become refractory to all medical therapies. As the liver continues to fail, hepatic encephalopathy worsens, ascites continue to accumulate, and other complications progress. Chacexia and muscle wasting cannot be halted, no matter how many nutrients the patient receives. Kidney function may gradually fail and hepatorenal syndrome may develop.

In these very advanced cases of cirrhosis, also known as end-stage liver disease, only liver transplantation can save the patient's life.

Liver transplantation should be considered as a "life insurance policy" for individuals with chronic hepatitis C. Most individuals with chronic hepatitis C will *not* need liver transplantation. But if they do, it can save their lives. The goal of liver transplantation in end-stage liver disease is to replace the patient's liver just before the complications of cirrhosis become refractory to medical treatment. In ideal situations, this can be estimated. In many cases, however, there is considerable uncertainty as to how soon the complications of cirrhosis and liver failure will become immediately life threatening. For this reason, patients with cirrhosis and one or more of its complications should probably be evaluated at a center for liver transplantation at least two years before the doctor anticipates that the condition will deteriorate and medical treatment will no longer be satisfactory.

The most important aspect of liver transplantation for most patients with cirrhosis from chronic hepatitis C is for their doctors to know when to refer them to a transplantation center for evaluation. Good medical judgment is necessary, and the decision is not always easy. In cirrhosis, deterioration is usually gradual, and the doctor must decide at what time, during many years of follow-up, referral to a transplantation center is indicated. When complications of cirrhosis cannot be controlled medically, referral to a liver transplantation center is clearly indicated. These complications include worsening hepatic encephalopathy, refractory ascites, and difficulty in controlling bleeding from gastric or esophageal varices. Cachexia, or generalized wasting, sometimes becomes an unstoppable complication of cirrhosis and transplantation should be performed before such patients literally "waste away." Other important parameters to consider include the blood albumin concentration, blood bilirubin concentration, and prothrombin time. A low blood albumin concentration, rising blood bilirubin concentration, and prolonged prothrombin time indicate deterioration in liver function.

There are a few reasons *not* to refer a patient with end-stage liver disease for transplantation. Virtually no center will transplant patients who are actively abusing or dependent on alcohol or other drugs. Such patients should first, or at least concurrently, be referred to a rehabilitation facility. Few centers will perform transplantation in patients over seventy years of age. At present, most centers will not transplant individuals with HIV infection; however, a few might. Patients with metastatic cancer or other terminal diseases are usually ineligible for liver transplantation. *If a doctor cannot determine if one of his or her patients is eligible for liver transplantation, he or she should contact a liver specialist at the nearest transplantation center to find out.*

For patients with end-stage liver disease who are referred for liver transplantation, the process can be divided into three phases: (1) pretransplant, (2) transplant, and (3) posttransplant. The actual transplant surgery is brief compared to the pretransplant and posttransplant periods. Patients generally have the most anxiety and questions during the pretransplant phase. The posttransplant phase lasts for the rest of the patient's lifetime.

On their first visit to a liver transplantation center, patients will usually be seen first by a *hepatologist* or medical liver specialist. During the first visit, a transplant surgeon may also see the patient, perhaps just to be introduced. The hepatologist will take a complete medical history, review past medical records, and perform a physical examination. The hepatologist should answer the patient's and family members' questions. The hepatologist will order a battery of blood tests, some routine, some specific to the case, and some particularly relevant to the transplant evaluation, such as blood typing.

At the first visit to a liver transplantation center, the patient and family members will likely meet a nurse coordinator who specializes in the care of patients undergoing organ transplantation. Throughout the pretransplantation evaluation, the patient will probably get to know the nurse coordinators the best of all members of the transplant team; often they are the first people the patient calls with questions or problems. These nurses, as the name indicates, coordinate all the multiple tests, doctor visits, and special procedures that patients being evaluated for liver transplantation require.

At the time of the initial consultation, the patient and family members may meet with a financial counselor. Liver transplantation is a very expensive procedure. The financial counselor will obtain detailed information about the patient's insurance coverage. Many major insurance policies, including federal and state programs such as Medicaid and Medi-Cal, will cover the costs. Problems sometimes occur with uninsured patients. The financial counselor may help such patients apply for benefits, or try to help arrange coverage for other expensive aspects of transplantation, such as the costs of medicine after the procedure.

A patient undergoing a liver transplant evaluation will require several radiological tests. A chest x-ray, liver ultrasound, and CAT scan will almost always be performed. The CAT scan will be done to measure the volume of the liver. This is important because a small person will need a small donor liver and a larger person will need a larger liver. Other radiological procedures or scans may also be performed as indicated.

As part of the transplant evaluation, the patient will see several different doctors and health professionals. Many patients, especially older ones, will see a cardiologist for an evaluation of their hearts. Cigarette smokers and patients with lung diseases will see a pulmonologist, or medical lung specialist. Patients with kidney problems will be evaluated by a nephrologist, or kidney specialist. Most patients will see a psychiatrist, especially those with a history of alcohol or drug abuse. All patients, and usually their family members as well, will frequently see a social worker for help dealing with stress and other issues associated with liver transplantation. Patients may also have to see a dentist to remove teeth that are decaying and could become a source of infection. Visits to other specialists or subspecialists may be scheduled as necessary.

Once the patient has undergone the necessary tests and has been evaluated by members of the transplant team and other physicians, the case is discussed in a meeting with members of the transplant team. The various doctors, nurse coordinators, financial counselors, and social workers may be asked to provide their impressions of the patient's suitability for organ transplantation. After the discussion, the group as a whole decides whether or not the patient is eligible.

If the patient is deemed eligible, he or she is put on the waiting list, or listed. Sometimes, for various medical, psychological, or social reasons, the team decides that the patient is not a transplant candidate.

Rarely, patients are not listed because they may not need the procedure. Such patients will usually be followed by their primary care doctors, sometimes in consultation with the transplant team, and reevaluated at a later date if their conditions deteriorate. Some patients are deemed ineligible for liver transplantation because other serious illnesses, such as cancer, AIDS, or heart disease, are identified during the pretransplant evaluation. Psychological and social problems, such as active illicit drug use or alcohol abuse, may also lead to a patient not being listed. Patients actively abusing drugs or alcohol will usually be turned down but may be offered another chance in the future if they demonstrate at least six months of abstinence and participation in programs such as Alcoholics Anonymous.

Once a patient with liver disease is listed for transplantation, a waiting period begins. The patient generally waits until a suitable liver becomes available from a cadaveric donor—a person who dies and donates organs. In the United States, rules about who receives available organs are established by the United Network for Organ Sharing (UNOS). The waiting time will vary. Some patients who are not that sick yet may wait for a few years. Severely ill patients may receive livers within a few weeks. Livers are not allocated on a strict first-come, first-served basis; a combination of how long the patient has been on the waiting list and how sick he or she is determines when the transplant surgery will occur. Donor organs must match the recipient in blood type and size. For example, a small liver from a donor with type A blood will be transplanted into a small recipient with type A blood. Some centers will perform "split liver" transplantation, in which parts of one donor liver are given to two different recipients. To some extent, the type of liver that becomes available will determine when an individual will be transplanted. Most patients who are listed eventually receive livers and are successfully transplanted. Unfortunately, because of an overall shortage of organs, some patients, especially those referred late, may die before a liver becomes available for them.

When a suitable donor organ becomes available, the patient is either called at home or beeped on a pager and told to report to the hospital. If the patient is already hospitalized, he or she will be informed that it is time for surgery. The patient is then prepared for surgery and taken to the operating room. Liver transplantation is *orthotopic* in that the new liver is put in the same place as the old one. The trickiest part of the surgery is probably attaching the bile duct from the new liver to the recipient's bile duct that remains in place. A major complication of liver transplant surgery is bleeding. Patients who undergo liver transplantation often have massive blood loss. Transfusion of many units of red blood cells, fresh frozen plasma, and platelets may be necessary during surgery.

Some patients may undergo "living-related" liver transplantation once they are determined eligible for liver transplantation and placed on the waiting list for a donor organ. In these cases, instead of waiting for a cadaveric organ, a family member or close friend donates a part of his or her liver to transplant into the patient. Living-related liver transplantation should only be performed at a center with considerable experience in this procedure. Before surgery, both the patient and the donor must be aware of all the risks and benefits of the procedure. Once patients are approved for living-related transplantation and the donor agrees, the surgery can be performed when everyone is ready, after undergoing proper medical, psychological, and social evaluations.

After surgery, the patient is taken to a recovery room, then usually to the surgical intensive care unit. Most patients wake up within twenty-four hours after surgery while on a respirator. Some patients will need kidney dialysis for a few days after transplantation. Blood testing is performed regularly to make sure that the transplanted liver is functioning. Medications to prevent rejection of the transplanted liver are begun at surgery and continued thereafter. The concentrations of some of these medications in the blood are monitored closely, and the doses may have to be adjusted frequently. If all goes well, a patient can leave the hospital less than two weeks after liver transplantation. Sometimes, complications arise that require longer hospital stays or even retransplantation.

Complications directly resulting from surgery can occur in the immediate posttransplant period. These include bile leaks from the newly sewn-together bile ducts, which must be treated by placement of a drainage tube by ERCP (endoscopic retrograde cholangiopancreatography) or sometimes by surgery. Local wounds and more widespread infections can also occur after surgery. Bleeding can occur after any surgical procedure, and blood transfusions are frequently required after liver transplantation surgery. Postoperative surgical complications are usually treated successfully, but they sometimes require a return trip or two to the operating room to be repaired.

A major aspect of posttransplant care is to prevent organ rejection and infections. The recipient's immune system recognizes the transplanted liver as foreign and a strong immune response can occur against the transplanted organ that would destroy it. Without medications to suppress the immune system, known as immunosuppressive drugs, the grafted liver would be rejected. Virtually all patients receiving liver transplants will take either cyclosporine A (Sandimmune or Neoral) or tacrolimus (Prograft). Most patients will also take various combinations of prednisone, azathioprine (Imuran), and mycolphenolic mofetil (CellCept), which are agents that act by different mechanisms to suppress the immune system. These drugs are started during or right after transplant surgery. Each of these drugs has different side effects and doctors may change the drugs and adjust the doses depending on the patient's condition and adverse events. Drugs to prevent organ rejection are expensive, around $10,000 or more a year. Most important, *patients must take drugs to prevent rejection precisely as prescribed for the rest of their lives*. Failure to take these drugs can lead to severe rejection and certain death.

For a period of time after discharge from the hospital, patients will generally return to see a doctor on the transplant team once a week. During these visits, laboratory tests will be checked for evidence of rejection, hepatitis, or abnormal liver function. Liver biopsy may be necessary if these are suspected. Medications may be adjusted depending on the results of laboratory tests and side effects the patient experiences. If things remain stable, the frequency of follow-up visits will gradually decrease.

Rejection can occur anytime after liver transplantation. Abnormal blood test results are usually the first indication. Most episodes of rejection will be detected by increases in the blood ALT and AST activities. Rejection can only definitively be diagnosed by a liver biopsy. If blood testing suggests rejection, liver biopsy will be performed. The majority of patients will experience some rejection the first couple of weeks after liver transplantation. Most of these rejection episodes are mild or moderate and respond to intravenous steroids followed by a brief period of increased oral prednisone. Severe rejection episodes, or those not responding to steroids, are usually treated by intravenous administration of monoclonal antibodies against lymphocytes, the white blood cells that attack the transplanted organ. About 10 percent of patients who undergo liver transplantation develop rejection that does not respond to drugs. For these patients, retransplantation is the only available option.

Infection is another common and potentially dangerous complication after liver transplantation. Because the immune system is suppressed by antirejection drugs, posttransplant patients are at risk for infections that patients with normally functioning immune systems do not get. These include infection with *Pneumocystis carinii*, which causes pneumonia, and cytomegalovirus (CMV), which causes many problems including hepatitis in the new liver. Patients may take a combination of trimethoprim and sulfamethoxazole (Bactrim or Septra) to prevent *Pneumocystis carinii* pneumonia. Some centers use gancyclovir (Cytovene) to prevent CMV infection, which is also used to treat it. CMV infection can mimic rejection, and the two can usually only be differentiated by a liver biopsy. Many other infections can occur that do not cause problems in people with normal immune systems, including those by fungi, *Mycobacteria*, and other viruses such as herpes.

A special concern after liver transplantation for hepatitis C is that the original disease will occur in the new organ. In nearly all people with hepatitis C who undergo liver transplantation, the transplanted liver becomes infected with the hepatitis C virus. Fortunately, the degree of hepatitis is usually mild and the patient does well. However, severe and rapidly progressive hepatitis caused by the hepatitis C virus sometimes occurs in a transplanted liver. Liver biopsy must be performed to differentiate rejection or other problems from severe recurrent hepatitis C. Treatment with interferon alpha with or without ribavirin may be indicated if severe hepatitis C recurs in the new liver. This treatment should only be carried out by doctors at the transplantation center who have extensive experience in dealing with such patients.

The overall five-year survival rate for patients who undergo liver transplantation at most centers is about 90 percent. Many patients recover fully enough to return to productive lives at home and at work within a few months of surgery. Patients must continue to take their immunosuppressive and other drugs as prescribed and follow up regularly with their doctors. They should contact their doctors immediately if problems arise.

7

Living with Hepatitis C

THE DIAGNOSIS OF hepatitis C is *not* a death sentence. Make long-term plans. Enjoy life to the fullest. The odds are that you will live a long and productive life. This is the most important advice I can provide about living with hepatitis C!

Although the odds are against it, there is a chance that a person who lives with chronic hepatitis C for many years will some day develop the complications of cirrhosis. This is what scares most patients: the thought of what *could* happen to them. Many patients obsess over this. I therefore try to get patients with chronic hepatitis C to remember the following critical points:

- The majority of patients with chronic hepatitis C will live normal and long lives and die from something other than liver disease.
- Currently available treatments are beneficial in about half of all patients.
- Better treatments will undoubtedly be available in the future.
- Liver transplantation is a "life insurance policy." Although the majority of patients with chronic hepatitis C will not need liver transplantation, it is available to save your life.

The odds are in the patient's favor. Hepatitis C will *not* kill most people. Current treatments are good and better treatments are down the road. If necessary, liver transplantation can save one's life. This is true for just about every patient with chronic hepatitis C.

In *The Liver Disorders Sourcebook*, I identified uncertainty, fear, lack of information, and misinformation as the things that terrify most patients with any chronic liver disease, including hepatitis C. Many patients are uncertain about whether the disease will shorten their lives and live in fear that the disease will kill them. This uncertainty and fear can be difficult to overcome. Patients with such feelings should discuss them openly with their doctors. If your fear is excessive and interfering with your life, consultation with a psychiatrist, psychologist, or social worker may be indicated. There are also support groups to help patients with liver diseases.

Lack of information also leads to fear in many patients with chronic hepatitis C. I always say, again and again: Ask your doctor! If for some reason you do not trust your doctor, obtain a second opinion to alleviate your concerns or find a doctor whom you do trust. Remember, a doctor who examines you and knows your complete history is the only person who can provide precise prognostic information. Sources of general information, such as this book, can help educate you about your illness and enable more meaningful discussions with the doctor; however, sources of general information can *never* substitute for your doctor. The combination of general information and specific information about your particular case, which only your doctor can provide, will help reduce fear about having chronic hepatitis C.

Beware of misinformation. This is especially true when using the Internet. On the World Wide Web, anyone can look like an expert. Beware of Web sites with information on "new" or "miracle" cures for chronic hepatitis C. Use only reliable Internet resources, such as those created by medical schools or legitimate patient organizations. Use them as a complement, *not* a substitute, for good medical care. Never believe everything you read or hear about hepatitis C. Always do more research to determine if something you hear is true. In particular, be highly suspicious of claims about miraculous alternative remedies that doctors are not aware of. Believe me, if these remedies were truly groundbreaking, mainstream doctors and scientists would know about them. Remedies that have not been subjected to scientific scrutiny and tested in controlled clinical trials should *never* be considered as drugs or treatments. Many herbal or alternative remedies have not been shown to be safe for patients with chronic hepatitis C.

Medical Follow-Up and Cancer Screening

Patients with chronic hepatitis C should have regular medical follow-ups, whether or not they are candidates for drug treatment. They should periodically see their doctors even if a sustained response is achieved after treatment. Even individuals without symptoms, normal blood ALT and AST activities, and minimal inflammation on liver biopsies should follow up with their doctors. The progression of the disease is difficult to predict; for this reason, a patient with chronic hepatitis C should be examined by a doctor at least once a year. Patients with cirrhosis and its complications should see their doctors more frequently and as needed if their conditions worsen. A complete physical examination should be performed at least once a year, and blood tests should be checked for possible deterioration in liver function.

Chronic hepatitis C virus is associated with the development of hepatocellular carcinoma (primary liver cancer). Almost all patients with chronic hepatitis C who develop cancer also have cirrhosis. However, there are a few reports of liver cancer in noncirrhotic patients with chronic hepatitis C. An important aspect of follow-up care of a patient with chronic hepatitis C is screening for hepatocellular carcinoma. There are no strict guidelines regarding frequency, and no data exist on overall efficacy and cost effectiveness of such screening. A National Institutes of Health Consensus Statement on hepatitis C, "Management of Hepatitis C," recommended that periodic screening for hepatocellular carcinoma be performed.

Cancer screening involves ultrasound studies to look for tumors and blood testing for alpha-fetoprotein, a marker of hepatocellular carcinoma. The blood alpha-fetoprotein concentration is elevated in about 85 percent of patients with hepatocellular carcinoma, and an increasing blood concentration may suggest the development of a small tumor. Patients with cirrhosis should probably have more frequent cancer screening than those without cirrhosis. Since conclusive data on the efficacy and cost effectiveness of cancer screening in patients with chronic hepatitis C do not exist, it is up to the individual doctor to determine how frequently periodic screening should be performed. Probably once a year for patients with cirrhosis is prudent. Some doctors may recommend twice a year.

The definitive diagnosis of hepatocellular carcinoma is made by biopsy. If an ultrasound scan indicates a possible tumor, a biopsy should generally be performed. Usually, the liver with a suspected tumor is biopsied by a radiologist under CAT scan or ultrasound guidance. Sometimes, it is biopsied using a laparoscope, a fiber-optic instrument that is inserted into the abdomen. Rarely, open surgical biopsy is necessary.

Hepatocellular carcinoma may be curable by surgery if the tumor is small. Surgery may not be possible in individuals with advanced cirrhosis. If surgery is contemplated, extensive presurgical evaluation by CAT scanning, magnetic resonance scanning, and angiography (injection of dye into the hepatic artery followed by x-rays) is required. Some patients with cirrhosis and small hepatocellular carcinomas (less than 5 centimeters in diameter and confined to the liver) may be treated by liver transplantation. For large tumors, or cancer that has spread beyond the liver, chemotherapy, ligating (tying) or embolization (clotting) of the hepatic artery, alcohol injection into the tumor, or radiation may relieve symptoms and prolong life, but these procedures are not curative. Patients may also opt for enrollment in clinical trials using experimental procedures.

The prognosis after treatment of hepatocellular carcinoma depends on the size of the tumor and the extent to which the liver is already damaged by cirrhosis. For patients with hepatocellular carcinomas that are deemed to be surgically resectable, the five-year survival rate after surgery is 10 to 30 percent. For patients with hepatocellular carcinomas in whom complete surgical removal of the tumor is not possible, the five-year survival rate is about 1 percent. Most patients with hepatocellular carcinomas that have spread beyond the liver survive for only a few months. Patients with advanced cirrhosis generally do poorly after surgical resection and should be considered for possible liver transplantation if the tumors are small and have not spread. At the present time, conclusive data are lacking on survival rates after liver transplantation for small tumors. United States government programs such as Medicare will cover the cost of liver transplantation for hepatocellular carcinomas that are less than 5 centimeters.

Safe Alcohol Use in Patients with Chronic Hepatitis C

Many liver specialists argue that patients with chronic hepatitis C should consume *no* alcohol. My personal feeling, given the lack of data from well-controlled, forward-looking studies, is that patients with chronic hepatitis C should limit their alcohol intake to no more than a few drinks a few times a week. A couple of glasses of wine occasionally with a nice dinner, a beer at a ball game, or an occasional cocktail at a party will probably not be detrimental for the person with chronic hepatitis C. Drinking becomes problematic if it takes place on a regular daily basis. Patients with chronic hepatitis C certainly should not exceed a limit of two drinks a day and should probably keep their alcohol intake below this amount. The man who taught me how to be a hepatologist, the late Dr. Fenton Schaffner, used to tell his patients: "You can drink as long as you drink only the good stuff." A glass of good wine or a fine cocktail once in a while probably won't hurt. An entire bottle of wine, a quart of liquor, or a six-pack of beer on a regular basis will definitely cause problems. Patients with alcohol abuse or dependency disorders, however, must completely abstain from alcohol.

Patients with Hepatitis C and Alcohol and Drug Abuse

Individuals with chronic hepatitis C who are actively abusing alcohol or other drugs present a special problem. The social and psychological issues of patients who are substance abusers make their priorities quite different. Alcohol is the number one cause of liver disease in the Western world. In those same countries, injection drug use is a major risk factor for hepatitis C. For these reasons, a large number of patients with chronic hepatitis C also have alcohol and drug use disorders.

For patients with active substance use disorders, the top priority is to deal with the substance disorder. I cannot emphasize this enough. It goes for all alcohol and drug abusers, including those with chronic hepatitis C. Some general guidelines for all alcohol or substance abusers are:

Rehabilitation. Many individuals with drug or alcohol abuse or dependency disorders require inpatient rehabilitation. Rehabilitation is usually a one-month voluntary stay in a facility where intensive treatment is directed at the substance disorder.

Alcoholics Anonymous and Narcotics Anonymous. Alcoholics Anonymous (AA) is an informal society of more than two million recovering alcoholics in the United States, Canada, and other countries. These men and women meet in local groups, which range in size from a handful in some localities to many hundreds in larger communities. Narcotics Anonymous (NA) is a similar society for individuals with other drug abuse or dependency disorders. *Anybody can contact AA or NA. You do not need a referral.*

Concurrent medical care. The sick person with a drug or alcohol abuse or dependency disorder will also need medical care for other conditions while in a rehabilitation program or participating in AA or NA meetings. Such patients should regularly see a doctor who understands their treatment needs. Many rehabilitation programs also offer medical services. Some patients with substance disorders may also benefit from psychiatric care. Such patients should ask their primary care physician or liver specialist about referral to a psychiatrist, perhaps one with a special interest in substance abuse disorders.

Family support. Family members and friends should be supportive of an individual's commitment to treat a substance use disorder. If family members or friends are having a difficult time with a loved one who abuses alcohol, they can contact Al-Anon, a worldwide organization that offers a self-help recovery program for families and friends of alcoholics, whether or not the alcoholic seeks help or even recognizes the existence of a drinking problem. Al-Anon has a division called Alateen for younger family members of alcohol abusers.

The patient with chronic hepatitis C and a substance use disorder has at least two problems to deal with. You cannot address one and not the other. Such patients require medical care and in many cases psychiatric treatment and benefit from participation in programs such as AA or NA. In addition, the needs of patients with chronic hepatitis C are also relevant to these individuals. Most important, individuals with substance use disorders, and their doctors, family members, and friends, must realize that these disorders are almost always more serious than chronic hepatitis C.

Use of Other Drugs and Medications in Hepatitis C

Patients with chronic hepatitis C can generally use drugs prescribed by their doctors or over-the-counter medications just like any other person. Until the complications of cirrhosis develop, the liver generally functions normally and metabolizes drugs appropriately. Naturally, any patient, whether or not he or she has hepatitis C, should follow the instructions of his or her doctor regarding the use of prescription medications and the instructions on the labels of over-the-counter drugs.

Patients with cirrhosis, for whom liver function may be compromised, should be especially careful. Many drugs are metabolized in the liver, and dose adjustments of some drugs may be necessary. Such patients should consult their doctors before taking any medication, including those sold over the counter. *When in doubt, any person should contact his or her doctor with questions about medications.*

Vaccination for Hepatitis A and B

Some studies suggest that patients with chronic hepatitis C are at an increased risk of serious or life-threatening illness if they contact hepatitis A. It is not entirely clear if all individuals with chronic hepatitis C should be vaccinated against hepatitis A; however, it may be prudent. Patients should consult their doctors.

Hepatitis A is spread primarily by eating contaminated food or drinking contaminated water. Uncooked shellfish and salads are frequent vehicles of transmission. Cold cuts, fruits, fruit juices, milk, and vegetables have also been implicated in various outbreaks. Hepatitis A is more common in underdeveloped parts of the world with poor sanitary conditions. Travelers to such regions are at an increased risk for infection. Travelers to parts of the world where hepatitis A is common, especially those with chronic hepatitis C, should be vaccinated against hepatitis A. The United States Centers for Disease Control and Prevention in Atlanta, Georgia (on the Internet at www.cdc.gov), provide recommendations for travelers to specific parts of the world.

Hepatitis A vaccines provide long-term protection against the disease. Two shots are administered at six- to twelve-month intervals. Before travel, the first dose should be given at least four weeks before the trip. This usually provides protection for a short duration, but a booster is necessary six to twelve months later for long-term protection. People who have been previously infected with the hepatitis A virus are generally immune to another infection and episode of hepatitis A. Immune individuals have serum IgG antibodies against the hepatitis A virus that can be detected by blood testing. Such people do not need to be vaccinated.

The hepatitis B virus is spread in many of the same ways as the hepatitis C virus. Effective vaccines against the hepatitis B virus are available. Most current preparations contain hepatitis B surface antigen, which is manufactured using recombinant DNA technology. Three shots are needed in most individuals to assure long-term immunity. After the initial shot of vaccine, a second shot is given one month later, and a third shot six months after that. The large majority of individuals respond to three shots with the development of antibodies to the surface of the virus. Elderly individuals, or individuals with chronic diseases, are less likely to respond to vaccination for hepatitis B.

At present, universal vaccination against hepatitis B is recommended for all children. For adults, those who are at high risk of exposure to hepatitis B virus should be vaccinated. Such individuals include health care workers, household contacts of individuals with hepatitis B, sexual partners of individuals with chronic hepatitis B, possibly all sexually promiscuous individuals, and people from Western countries who will reside for extended periods of time in parts of the world where hepatitis B virus infection is endemic, such as southeast Asia and north Africa.

Pregnancy and Hepatitis C

Should a woman with chronic hepatitis C become pregnant? In young women with chronic hepatitis C without cirrhosis, the risk during pregnancy is low and probably not increased compared to otherwise healthy women. Of course, the mother and father must realize that there is a risk of passing on the hepatitis C virus to their baby. This risk appears to be less than 5 percent based on the results of most studies. This consideration aside, pregnancy is probably not a very high-risk condition for patients with chronic hepatitis C who do not have cirrhosis. Most young women with chronic hepatitis C who want to get pregnant can do so safely.

Women who are being treated for hepatitis C with ribavirin should *not* get pregnant during or soon after treatment. It is also recommended that men who are taking ribavirin should *not* impregnate their female sexual partners. Sexually active individuals who are taking ribavirin should use a safe and effective method of contraception. If a woman gets pregnant while either she or her sexual partner is taking ribavirin or very soon after stopping it, she should contact her doctor immediately.

The risks during pregnancy are increased in women with cirrhosis, even if they do not have clinical complications. In women with clinical complications of cirrhosis, pregnancy can be life threatening to both the mother and the fetus. Most women with very advanced cirrhosis are infertile, so pregnancy is not an issue. Elective abortion should be considered as an option in instances when the life of the mother and fetus are at risk. Women with cirrhosis who are contemplating pregnancy should discuss the issue with their doctors and perhaps also see a specialist in high-risk pregnancies. When pregnant, care from an obstetrician with experience in high-risk pregnancies will usually be necessary.

Children with Hepatitis C

Depending on their age and sophistication, children will have different degrees of insight into their medical conditions. *What is most important for parents to realize is that children with chronic hepatitis C should be treated like all other kids!* They should go to school, play, and participate in sports. Most will have long and normal lives and probably not suffer from complications of cirrhosis. Some studies in fact suggest that people infected with the hepatitis C virus very early in their lives have less progressive disease.

What about treatment for children? Several studies have looked at interferon alpha-based therapies in children with chronic hepatitis C and more are under way. It is still not entirely clear when children should be treated. Ribavirin should not be given to very young children as it may cause developmental defects. Parents should discuss treatment of their child's chronic hepatitis C with their pediatricians, and consult a pediatric liver specialist as appropriate. Children will benefit the most from ongoing research that will ultimately lead to more effective drugs.

Support Groups

Many patients with chronic hepatitis C seek out support groups to discuss their lives and their problems with other patients. There are many such groups, some mainstream and some alternative. With the growth of the Internet, there are countless chat rooms, groups, foundations, and agencies devoted to hepatitis C. One should be careful as some of these organizations propagate dangerous ideas and false information about the disease and its treatments. Following are two support groups for patients with hepatitis C that I feel are reputable. I have also included information on AA and NA for those with alcohol or drug abuse problems.

American Liver Foundation
75 Maiden Lane, Suite 603
New York, NY 10038
1-800-GO LIVER (465-4837)
www.liverfoundation.org

Hepatitis Foundation International
30 Sunrise Terrace
Cedar Grove, NJ 07009-1423
(201) 239-1035 or 1-800-891-0707
www.hepfi.org

Alcoholics Anonymous (AA) World Services, Inc.
P.O. Box 459
New York, NY 10163
(212) 870-3400
www.alcoholics-anonymous.org

Narcotics Anonymous (NA) World Services
P.O. Box 9999
Van Nuys, CA 91409
(818) 773-9999
www.na.org

8

Selecting the Right Doctor

An important choice for anyone with a chronic illness is selecting the right doctor or doctors. This is sometimes a daunting challenge, especially in this age of HMOs, PPOs, and other forms of managed care. In my opinion, three of the most critical things about selecting a doctor when you have a chronic illness are:

1. Finding one with knowledge and experience about your condition.
2. Finding one with the time and ability to explain things to you.
3. Finding one with whom you can communicate comfortably.

This sounds easy, but it can be quite complex. Sometimes the most knowledgeable experts are in academic medical centers and spend so much time on research and teaching that they have little time to talk to patients. In many cases, a person's health insurance will not cover certain specialists. In many cases, it is difficult to find a physician who has time to explain things while being forced to see a quota of patients each day. Some doctors, no matter how smart or accessible they are, just don't hit it off with some patients. This last issue is often dependent more on personality than competence but is still very important.

Most patients with chronic hepatitis C will have at least two doctors. The first will be their primary care doctor, the second will be the liver specialist—a *gastroenterologist* or *hepatologist*. Increasingly, infectious disease specialists will also treat patients with chronic hepatitis C, and a gastroenterologist or hepatologist may only be called on for liver biopsy. Some patients with chronic hepatitis C may need other specialists, for example, a psychiatrist if depression or substance abuse are issues. The primary care doctor and other specialists should work together in the patient's overall care. The primary care doctor will remain responsible for the patient's overall health care. The liver specialist will devote his or her effort primarily to the evaluation and treatment of chronic hepatitis C. Other specialists, if necessary, will focus on other specific problems.

The Primary Care Doctor

A diagnosis of chronic hepatitis C in adults is often made by the patient's primary care doctor, usually a family practitioner or internist. In the case of children, the primary care doctor is usually a family practitioner or pediatrician. Most primary care doctors in the United States and other developed countries should know how to diagnose chronic hepatitis C, or at least suspect the diagnosis. They will know to test for hepatitis C if a patient is found to have abnormal blood ALT or AST activities, usually as a result of blood testing for other reasons, for example, as part of a life or health insurance physical. Most primary care doctors will also know which of their patients with risk factors should be screened for hepatitis C, and patients should tell their primary care doctors if they have such risk factors. If a blood test for hepatitis C comes back positive, the primary care doctor will generally refer the patient to a specialist for further evaluation.

Most patients will be followed by their primary care doctors for the long term. If referral to a specialist is indicated, the primary care doctor should continue to follow the patient along with the specialist. The primary care doctor will be the person you contact for other medical problems, and he or she should be familiar with the treatment you may be receiving from the specialist. The primary care doctor should be able to answer your questions and help you understand what the specialist recommends and discuss your overall health with the specialist when deciding certain issues, such as your suitability for treatment with certain medications.

Is your primary care doctor competent? Internal medicine, pediatrics, and family practice all have their respective specialty boards. In order to receive board certification in these specialties, the doctor must undergo appropriate training and pass an examination given by a specialty board. A first step in determining the qualifications of your primary care doctor is to establish if he or she is board certified (having passed the specialty examination) or board eligible (having completed the necessary training to take the examination) in his or her specialty.

The Liver Specialist

For further evaluation, specialized procedures, and possible treatment, most primary care doctors will refer patients with chronic hepatitis C to *gastroenterologists*. Gastroenterologists are internists or pediatricians who complete specialty training in internal medicine or pediatrics. After completing specialty training, they usually do an additional three years of fellowship training in the subspecialty of gastroenterology. Most of this training focuses on diseases of the gastrointestinal track, primarily those of the esophagus, stomach, small intestine, colon, and rectum. Part of the training of all gastroenterology fellows is also focused on the diagnosis and treatment of liver diseases. There are subspecialty boards in gastroenterology, and although any doctor can call him- or herself a gastroenterologist, you can determine if yours has actually had adequate training in this field by asking if he or she is board certified or board eligible in gastroenterology.

In clinical practice, the majority of gastroenterologists devote most of their time to diseases of the colon, stomach, esophagus, and intestines. Some gastroenterologists take a special interest in hepatology, which is the study of liver diseases. Gastroenterologists who see a reasonable number of patients with liver diseases and are skilled in their diagnosis and treatment are often referred to as *hepatologists*. Some doctors who never formally trained in gastroenterology study liver diseases during their careers and become hepatologists. Internists and pediatricians who subspecialize in hepatology only (not gastroenterology) are usually only found at academic medical centers closely affiliated with medical schools.

There is no official subspecialty board in hepatology. It is therefore sometimes difficult to determine if doctors who call themselves hepatologists are actually experts in liver diseases. A doctor who is a full-time faculty member at a major medical school and considered to be a hepatologist is probably a legitimate one. Many such doctors will have published papers in peer-reviewed journals in the area of liver diseases. I do not mean pieces on the Internet, in "throwaway" medical journals, or even a book like this one, but scholarly articles in medical journals, which are reviewed by experts before they are published. In the United States, membership in the American Association for the Study of Liver Diseases (AASLD), a professional society, usually—but not always—indicates some expertise in hepatology.

The liver specialist should take a complete history and perform a physical examination the first time he or she sees you. The specialist may order additional blood tests. In the case of chronic hepatitis C, the gastroenterologist or hepatologist will frequently perform a liver biopsy. After reviewing all data, this doctor will suggest a treatment decision, usually in conjunction with the patient and the primary care doctor. The liver specialist will prescribe the treatment and follow the patient during treatment. As mentioned, some infectious disease specialists are starting to treat patients with chronic hepatitis C. This is especially true for those with concurrent HIV infection.

A patient with cirrhosis and complications may require more intensive care from a liver specialist. Those with significant complications of cirrhosis or end-stage liver disease ultimately need referral to a center where liver transplantation is performed, unless the patient is too old or has a concurrent condition that excludes liver transplantation. Liver transplantation centers have medical and pediatric liver specialists who have extensive expertise in the treatment of patients with end-stage liver disease. Liver transplantation centers also have surgeons who subspecialize in performing liver transplantation and other aspects of liver surgery. Such centers have doctors in a wide range of specialties and subspecialties who handle problems that may occur in patients with end-stage liver disease or after liver transplantation.

How to Find a Liver Specialist

How does a patient find a gastroenterologist or hepatologist knowledgeable in the care of patients with chronic hepatitis C? Usually the best source for a referral is the patient's primary care doctor, who will know the local and regional specialists and subspecialists in most areas of medicine.

What if your primary care doctor does not know a liver specialist? Or what if you do not like the specialist recommended by your primary care doctor? Some organizations keep track of medical specialists. Several publications found in public libraries list board-certified medical specialists. The American Liver Foundation, a national nonprofit health organization dedicated to preventing, treating, and curing liver diseases, has several local chapters that maintain lists of liver specialists in their regions. You can contact the American Liver Foundation (on the Internet at www.liverfoundation.org or at 1-800-GO LIVER) or the local chapter for the names of these specialists.

Some patients want to see an expert on chronic hepatitis C, even just once for a second-opinion consultation. Usually, the leading specialists and researchers are full-time faculty members at medical schools. Before seeing such a doctor, a patient should ask if it is really necessary. The special expertise of doctors at an academic medical center is not always necessary for most patients with chronic hepatitis C. For some patients, a one-time, second-opinion consultation with a specialist at a leading medical center, however, may help put their minds at ease by confirming the suggestions and recommendations of their regular doctors. Specialists at academic medical centers may also be able to enroll interested patients in appropriate clinical trials or other research protocols.

At medical centers with active research programs in liver diseases, there will usually be several specialists who devote most of their time to caring for patients with liver diseases. If you live near a leading medical school, and your insurance will cover the costs, you can usually call for referral to a specialist. Some will have phone numbers for referral services. Many patients do not know this, but the best way to find a medical subspecialist is to call the appropriate academic division directly. For example, if you are an adult with chronic hepatitis C, you can find the phone number for the Division of Gastroenterology or Division of Digestive and Liver Diseases in the Department of Medicine at a nearby medical school. For a child, the similar division in the Department of Pediatrics can be contacted. You will very likely find someone there who can direct you to a specialist for your problem. Academic divisions and departments at medical schools also often have Internet Web sites with doctor referral information. Remember, however, to exercise caution when looking for a doctor on the Internet since *any* doctor (or layperson, for that matter) can advertise their practices to look like world-renowned medical research institutions.

Problems with Managed Care

Many patients complain that their HMO doctors do not know enough about hepatitis C or that their HMO will not let them see a specialist. The validity of such complaints depends upon the particular managed care organization. Some HMOs are excellent and have a broad range of specialists accessible to their members. Some, frankly, do not. Most good managed care organizations will have a gastroenterologist who can adequately evaluate and care for patients with chronic hepatitis C. Most will also have a mechanism in place for referral to a liver transplantation program if necessary.

I do not know exactly how to help a patient who perceives that his or her HMO doctor is not qualified to undertake the appropriate evaluation and provide adequate treatment for chronic hepatitis C. The best option is to insist and persist. Call the company's top management and insist that you see another specialist if you think it is appropriate. It is also possible to explore legal options in the rare instances when your HMO or insurance provider is prohibiting referral to a specialist for chronic hepatitis C.

Life comes before money. In some instances, it may be in your best interest to pay cash for a one-time, second-opinion consultation with a liver specialist that will not be covered by insurance or the managed care program. Odds are that you will be relieved to hear that your current doctor is doing things right. This will probably be worth the cost of one visit. If by chance you find out from an expert that your current doctor is not handling your problems correctly, a letter from a noted liver specialist at an academic institution explaining why you need different care *may* help in convincing your managed care providers to cover the cost of outside care.

9

Research and Hope for the Future

New Drugs Down the Road

The hepatitis C virus was discovered in 1989. In the dozen years since then, tremendous progress has been made in the diagnosis of chronic hepatitis C. Treatment, however, has only reached 50 percent efficacy. Research on the virus and the disease it causes has been slowed partly for the following two reasons:

1. It has not been possible to replicate the hepatitis C virus in cultured cells in the laboratory.
2. There is no small-animal model of hepatitis C; the smallest animals infected with the hepatitis C virus so far are humans and chimpanzees.

Despite these limitations, it is inevitable that better drugs for chronic hepatitis C will be available in the future, given the speed of scientific discovery in this new millennium. Although the hepatitis C virus cannot be cultured in the laboratory, scientists have developed subgenomic replicons in which a portion of the viral genome can be replicated in cells. They have also characterized in great detail most of the proteins of the hepatitis C virus and developed assays to examine their functions in vitro (outside of cells). Patients with chronic hepatitis C will directly benefit from all this scientific research.

This chapter explains potential new treatments for patients with chronic hepatitis C. Remember that this disease progresses slowly, so most patients will benefit from ongoing research before they develop serious complications.

Of course, nothing is guaranteed. Scientific advances often come as surprises. However, based on what has been learned about the hepatitis C virus and on other advances in the biomedical sciences, I will try to make some logical predictions about new treatments for patients with chronic hepatitis C.

Meet the New Drugs, Same as the Old Drugs

The next "new drugs" available to treat chronic hepatitis C are likely to be the same as the old drugs. Peginterferon alpha has recently been approved. The active agents in peginterferon alphas are the same old interferon alphas. By attaching the proteins to polyethylene glycol, the half-life of interferon alpha is prolonged in the body. More constant blood levels of interferon alpha are thus achieved with less frequent injections (usually once a week). Patients are therefore more likely to follow the prescribed drug regimen, which results in superior antiviral activity. Preparations of interferon alpha, with even longer half-lives than peginterferon, may be available in the future. At least one is currently in early-stage clinical testing. This is a recombinant fusion protein between albumin and interferon alpha. Data on its clinical efficacy are not yet available. It is also probable that other longer acting preparations of interferon alpha will be developed in the next few years. These will still be the same old interferon alphas, but the longer half-lives may further enhance patient compliance and efficacy of the drug. A potential concern if the patient suffers from side effects is that interferon alpha will remain in the body longer.

A drug known as VX-497, now in early clinical testing, is similar to ribavirin. The hope is that this drug and others like it will be more efficacious than ribavirin, without the side effect of hemolytic anemia.

In the near future, clinical research for chronic hepatitis C will focus largely on currently available drugs, or slightly different versions, administered in different ways. Duration and dosage will be tweaked to slightly improve efficacy, enhance compliance, and reduce side effects. Some studies will look at long-term maintenance interferon alpha for people who relapse when treatment is stopped. Others may look at high-dose, intensive short courses of interferon with and without ribavirin. It is unlikely that any of this near-term clinical research based on interferon alpha will lead to great breakthroughs. It will only lead to slight improvements over what is already available.

Specific Agents Against the Hepatitis C Virus

The next generation of breakthrough drugs will be those designed specifically to inhibit functions of the hepatitis C virus. To understand these drugs, it is important to explain a few critical steps in the life cycle of the hepatitis C virus (see Figure 9.1). All these steps are potential targets for antiviral drugs. Much more is known about some of these steps than others.

In step 1, the virus binds to a receptor or receptors on the cell surface. At present, the exact identities of the cell surface receptors for the hepatitis C virus are not known. One candidate receptor is a protein known as CD81, which binds to the viral envelope protein E2. Another candidate receptor is the LDL receptor, a protein that binds to certain complexes of cholesterol. However, it has not been rigorously proven that these proteins are actually the receptors that mediate viral entry into cells. This is technically difficult to prove, as a cell culture system for the hepatitis C virus does not exist.

After the hepatitis C virus binds to a cell surface receptor or receptors, it enters the cell. In step 2, the lipid envelope of the virus fuses with the cell membrane and the viral particles enter the cell. Based on what is known about other enveloped viruses such as HIV, this step likely involves a complex relationship between the viral envelope proteins and the cell surface receptor proteins. Once in the cell, the envelope is removed from the viral particles and the RNA is released (step 3). Very little is known about this uncoating step.

Figure 9.1 Life Cycle of the Hepatitis C Virus

The numbered points are potential targets for the development of antiviral drugs.

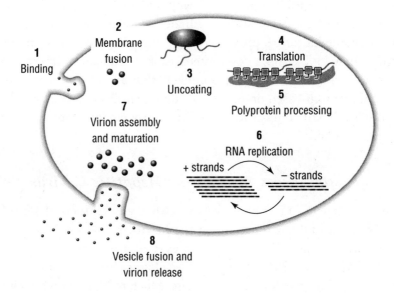

1. Virus binds to a receptor or receptors on the cell surface.
2. Enveloped virus fuses with the cell membrane and enters the cell.
3. Viral RNA is uncoated.
4. Viral RNA is translated to protein on host cell ribosomes.
5. Large viral polyprotein is cut into smaller proteins.
6. Viral RNA is replicated.
7. Mature viral particles are assembled.
8. Viral particles fuse with the cell membrane and are released.

As depicted in step 4, the hepatitis C viral RNA accesses the cell's ribosomes, the structure in which translation (protein synthesis) occurs. This step is mediated by an internal ribosome entry site (IRES), a highly conserved structure at the front end of the viral RNA. In contrast, most cellular RNAs bind to ribosomes through atoms attached to the front end of the RNA molecule, a chemical modification known as a 5' cap. After being synthesized, the large viral polyprotein is processed into smaller proteins (step 5). A cellular enzyme known as *signal peptidase* and two proteases, NS2 and

NS3, which are encoded by the viral RNA, catalyze this processing. After the viral proteins are synthesized, the viral RNA is replicated (step 6). The NS5B protein of the hepatitis C virus, which has RNA-directed RNA polymerase activity, catalyzes viral RNA replication. The viral NS3 helicase probably plays an important role in translation and replication, keeping the RNA in an accessible, unwound configuration.

After the viral RNA is replicated and protein synthesized, new viral particles are assembled in the cells (step 7). The mature viruses, or virions, ultimately fuse with the plasma membrane and are released (step 8). Little is known about how the hepatitis C virus is assembled. The fusion and release step may utilize the same cellular pathway as many other viruses and secreted proteins.

The steps in the hepatitis C virus life cycle that pharmaceutical companies are focusing on right now are polyprotein processing and RNA replication. A considerable amount of information is already available on the viral proteins that catalyze these processes. The three-dimensional structures of the hepatitis C virus NS3 helicase domain, the NS3 protease domain, the NS3 protease domain complexed with NS4A, and the NS5B RNA polymerase have all been determined by x-ray crystallography. Armed with this knowledge, pharmaceutical chemists can more readily design compounds that inhibit these functions. This method is called *rational drug design*. Rational drug design can be combined with combinatorial chemistry, in which libraries of thousands or more structurally similar molecules are synthesized and tested to identify the ones that inhibit the target best. These "hits" can be improved on and ultimately tested in chimpanzees and then possibly humans. It is likely that in the current decade, hepatitis C virus protease inhibitors, helicase inhibitors, and RNA polymerase inhibitors will be tested in trials to treat patients with hepatitis C. My guess is that combinations of these specific antiviral drugs will some day be the standard of care for treating patients.

Another potential drug target of the hepatitis C virus is the IRES of its RNA. The hepatitis C virus IRES is a unique RNA structure probably not shared by host cell RNAs. Various methods to identify compounds that bind to the hepatitis C virus RNA IRES are being used. The viral RNA is the target of other potential drugs in addition to IRES inhibitors. Molecules known as ribozymes—catalytic RNAs that splice other RNAs—are currently being tested to treat hepatitis C. Ribozymes have been synthesized that recognize parts of the hepatitis C virus RNA molecule that are found in all hepatitis C genotypes. These molecular parts are called *conserved sequences*. The ribozymes cut the RNA at that point, hence inactivating it. They have been shown to work in the test tube and are currently in early human clinical trials. "Antisense" RNA molecules, synthetic RNAs that are complementary in sequence to the viral RNA, are also being tested. These molecules recognize and bind to the viral RNA, and then cause it to be degraded by certain cellular enzymes. Drugs that bind to hepatitis C viral RNA, or to the core protein with which it associates, could also potentially block viral assembly and maturation.

The binding of the hepatitis C virion to its cell membrane receptor, and the subsequent membrane fusion that allows for entry into the cell, are also potential targets for specific antiviral drugs. Drugs that bind to the two candidate hepatitis C virus receptors, CD81 and LDL receptor, can potentially be developed into inhibitors of viral binding to cells. Further research is needed, however, to confirm that these proteins are receptors or to identify the actual ones. The technical drawback in developing drugs to inhibit virus binding and entry is the lack of a cell culture system to test for viral entry. Various small molecules are also being tested that block the fusion of the viral lipid envelope with the cell membrane after the virus has bonded with surface receptors.

One cannot accurately predict the adverse event profile of a given drug until it is tested in humans. Drugs that are well designed against specific targets of the hepatitis C virus may still prove to have side effects. However, they are likely to be more effective and better tolerated than currently available interferon alpha-based treatments for hepatitis C. As most of these drugs are still in preclinical development, the time line from the laboratory to the clinic is likely to be several years. Once these promising agents are ready for human testing, clinical trials in patients will be necessary to show efficacy and safety before approval by regulatory agencies such as the FDA. These trials will take several years to conduct.

Drugs That Affect the Immune Response Against the Virus

Several drugs known as immune modifiers or immunomodulators, which alter the immune response, are also being tested for chronic hepatitis C. Some are being studied along with interferon alpha. These drugs alter the immune response against liver cells infected with the virus. Their mechanisms of action are poorly understood. Compounds of this type currently being tested in humans include thymosin-alpha-1 and histamine dihydrocholoride. These drugs may add to the efficacy of interferon alpha.

Therapeutic vaccines are also being developed to enhance the immune response against the hepatitis C virus. In contrast to a preventive vaccine, a therapeutic vaccine is administered to individuals already infected to stimulate the immune system to fight the infection. Preventive vaccines for hepatitis C are also under development. Because the virus mutates rapidly, development of an effective preventive vaccine is a huge challenge. If and when an effective preventive vaccine is developed, it would truly be revolutionary and have the potential to eradicate the hepatitis C virus.

Drugs That Affect the Liver's Response to Injury

Chronic hepatitis can lead to fibrosis and ultimately cirrhosis, the dreaded complication of hepatitis C. Nearly all the serious complications of chronic hepatitis C result from cirrhosis. For this reason, drugs to prevent fibrosis and cirrhosis could be of great benefit. Recent data suggest that fibrosis, and perhaps even early cirrhosis, may be reversible to some extent.

Unfortunately, very little is known about why the liver becomes fibrotic in response to chronic hepatitis. Furthermore, it is not known why some individuals infected with the hepatitis C virus develop significant fibrosis or cirrhosis while others never do.

Increasing scientific effort is being devoted to the study of liver fibrosis in response to injury, and exciting new drugs to prevent it will hopefully be available some day.

Stem Cells

When a liver is severely cirrhotic and damaged beyond repair, the only hope today is liver transplantation. Considerable research is being devoted to the study of stem cells, undifferentiated cells such as those in the early embryo, which can be directed to form many different tissues of the body. In the past few years, investigators have shown that liver stem cells reside in the bone marrow. Theoretically, these bone marrow stem cells can be isolated and grown into hepatocytes and bile duct cells in the laboratory. Some animal studies have also shown that expression in liver cells of the enzyme telomerase, necessary to replicate chromosome ends, enhances their ability to regenerate. Although considerable practical challenges remain to be overcome, this early-stage research provides promise that liver transplantation may some day be a thing of the past.

Genomics

Research on hepatitis C will benefit from the recently completed human genome project. The entire sequence of DNA that makes up the human genome is now known to scientists. This information can be of great value in figuring out why some drugs work in some patients but not in others. Only about half of all patients achieve the desirable sustained response with the drugs currently available to treat hepatitis C. Similarly, treatment causes significant side effects in some patients while others tolerate it well. Some of the differences in antiviral response may have to do with the particular viral isolate infecting the patient. For example, genotype 1 isolates are more resistant to interferon alpha treatment than other genotypes. However, even among individuals infected with the same genotype virus, the response to treatment is highly variable. Most of this variability, as well as variability in side effects, is a result of different individuals' different genetic makeups.

Pharmacogenomics is the science of understanding the correlation between an individual's genetic makeup and response to a drug. The discipline is currently in its infancy but evolving rapidly. Pharmacogenomics aims to identify genetic markers that predict patients' responses to a drug. The genetic markers commonly assessed are known as single nucleotide polymorphisms (SNPs) and haplotypes. SNPs are changes at a single base of DNA between individuals. Haplotypes are linear arrays of slightly different forms of particular genes on a chromosome. By studying populations of patients and their responses to a drug, inheritance of a collection of SNPs or different haplotypes can be correlated with successful treatment, unsuccessful treatment, or the development of side effects. This knowledge can then be used to customize drug therapy for a particular patient based on first examining his or her DNA. An interesting place to start would be in determining which patients with chronic hepatitis C are likely to achieve a sustained response to interferon and which are likely to suffer significant side effects.

The same methods used in pharmacogenomics could also theoretically be used to predict a patient's prognosis. For example, inheritance of certain forms of certain genes may predispose a person with chronic hepatitis C to develop cirrhosis after many years. Other forms of genes may protect against the development of significant inflammation, fibrosis, or cirrhosis. Identification of such genes could lead to tests that predict who may have to be treated for chronic hepatitis and who may never develop cirrhosis. This would make the scary uncertainty associated with chronic hepatitis C a thing of the past.

Participation in Clinical Trials

Many patients with chronic hepatitis C want to be enrolled in studies or clinical trials. Potential subjects should realize that there is a broad range of clinical trials, from testing of new drugs for approval by the FDA or similar agencies in other countries to postmarketing trials.

There are several key players in a clinical trial. One is the sponsor, which is usually the pharmaceutical company that manufactures the drug. The sponsor provides the financial support for the trial and has a lot to gain if it is successful, such as approval of a new drug or more data supporting an approved drug's use. There may also be an outside monitor who oversees the trial. The study investigator and subinvestigators are the individuals who carry out the clinical trial. Study investigators are usually physicians who practice at academic medical centers and have appointments at medical schools. Some may be practitioners in private practice. The study investigators enroll patients, give the drugs, follow the patients, and obtain the data. There is also the Institutional Review Board (IRB), a committee composed of doctors and laypersons, such as members of the clergy, lawyers, ethicists, and other members of the community. The IRB reviews and approves the study protocol with the safety of the subjects being of paramount importance. *A person should never participate in a clinical trial that is not approved by an IRB.*

In the United States, a drug must undergo rigorous testing before the FDA approves it for use. The testing must prove *efficacy* and *safety*. When a pharmaceutical manufacturer wants to introduce a new drug, it must first go through several phases of clinical trials. The FDA must approve the start of each phase of testing. The FDA must also review data on an ongoing basis from the sponsor, especially reports of adverse events, and can stop the trials at any time.

In phase I trials, the drug is introduced to human subjects. This phase occurs after the drug has been tested in animals. For hepatitis C, animal testing usually means chimpanzees. Phase I trials involve only a small number of subjects and are done to study the pharmacokinetics, side effects, and safety of the drug. Phase I clinical trials are *not* intended to address efficacy of treatment of a disease. They may even be done in healthy volunteers.

If Phase I studies are completed without documented serious toxicity, Phase II clinical trials begin. These trials are designed to obtain additional safety data and to determine the preliminary effectiveness of the drug and what dose is likely to be optimal. Several hundred subjects are usually enrolled in Phase II clinical trials.

Phase III clinical trials are undertaken after Phase II studies have established that an experimental drug may indeed be safe and potentially effective in patients with the disease. In Phase III clinical trials, the new drug or treatment protocol is usually compared with an existing treatment or a placebo treatment. The study is usually double-blinded and randomized. *Double-blind* means that neither the investigator nor the patients know if they are receiving the study drug, an existing treatment, or a placebo. *Randomized* means that subjects are assigned by chance to receive either the study drug or the existing treatment or placebo. In this way, bias is removed from the trial. In Phase III clinical trials, subject groups can range from several hundred to several thousand. If Phase III clinical trials show safety and efficacy after the data are subjected to rigorous statistical analysis, the FDA may approve the drug for the disease it was tested against.

After FDA approval is gained, a new drug may continue to be tested in Phase IV trials after the substance is in widespread use. Many Phase IV trials provide useful new information on the drug's safety and its use in special populations. However, it is often after a drug is approved and on the market that potential study subjects should exercise caution when enrolling in a study. "Clinical trials" of approved drugs do not always need FDA approval. Some Phase IV studies provide little more than currently available treatment and money to doctors for prescribing the new drug. The reputations of the sponsor, investigator, and institution where the study is taking place are important to consider before enrolling in a study of any drug, including those that are already approved for general use.

In the best clinical studies, some of the patients will receive a new or experimental treatment and others will receive a placebo or the currently available treatment. These studies often provide patients with access to new and promising drugs before the FDA approves them. In addition, study investigators frequently, *but not always*, have more expertise regarding the disease being studied.

In the past several years, there has been a proliferation of clinical trials for chronic hepatitis C. Many are serious clinical trials designed by academic investigators or major pharmaceutical companies to get new drugs approved. Unfortunately, some studies of hepatitis C drugs are nothing more than marketing efforts by manufacturers to get doctors to use their products. Many of these studies are not studies at all, but merely programs in which pharmaceutical companies pay doctors to prescribe their products to a group of patients. Many studies of this kind are poorly designed and their results will never be published. In recent years, these pseudo-trials have proliferated, especially as more pharmaceutical companies have competing products on the market.

What to Ask Before Enrolling

There are several things that patients should ask before enrolling in a study for the treatment of chronic hepatitis C (or any disease for that matter).

> *Where is the study taking place?* Most studies that take place at medical schools or academic medical centers are probably legitimate. At these institutions, an IRB assures that the trial is safe and ethical. Caution should be exercised in enrolling in studies in private doctors' offices. Some are completely legitimate, but some use so-called central IRBs that are essentially private companies that approve studies. Although many are legitimate, it is not always clear if these "central IRBs" have the same standards as those at medical schools or hospitals. *Always obtain proof of IRB approval before consenting to be in a clinical study.*

> *Who is the study sponsor?* Some studies are funded by the National Institutes of Health or other government agencies and are likely to be very good studies, but these are few and far between. Most studies are sponsored and financially supported by pharmaceutical companies and can either be investigator-initiated or company-initiated. The distinction is usually who designs the study. Some of the company studies may be marketing programs that merely pay doctors to prescribe particular drugs. On the other hand, many company-designed studies are the first and best trials to test a new drug. *Be suspicious of company studies of a drug that is already approved for the indication being studied.*

Who is the principal investigator of the study? A study with a full-time faculty member at a medical school as principal investigator is more likely to be a better choice than a study conducted in the office of a doctor who does not have a medical school affiliation. *Always find out as much as you can about the principal investigator of the study.*

Ask your doctor! Never enroll in a clinical trial without first discussing it with your doctor.

Most studies of drugs for hepatitis C will not be of new drugs conducted by professors at the best medical schools. On the other hand, most studies will not be mere marketing efforts to induce doctors to prescribe particular drugs. They are usually something in between. Just remember to make sure that the study is IRB-approved. Do some homework to find out the reputations of the sponsor and the investigators. *And always check with your doctor before enrolling.*

10

Herbal and Alternative Treatments: Consumer Beware!

OUTSIDE THE BOUNDARIES of mainstream allopathic medicine is the world of alternative medicine. Among the many alternative treatments available are herbal remedies, aromatherapy, massage therapy, music therapy, macrobiotics, traditional Chinese medicines, gemstones, and homeopathy. It is beyond the scope of this book to discuss all of the alternative treatments for chronic hepatitis C.

First and foremost, *consumers of alternative medicines should beware!* Alternative treatments are not subject to the rigorous clinical trials that pharmaceutical drugs are subjected to prior to approval by the FDA or similar agencies in other countries. This means that not only have they *not* been shown to be effective by currently accepted scientific standards, many have *not* been proven to be safe. There should be a sound scientific basis for the effectiveness of *any* substance, including herbs, to treat a disease or condition. Before a compound can be considered to be an effective drug in humans, it must be tested in clinical trials. The gold-standard clinical trial is a randomized, double-blind, placebo-controlled trial, as discussed in Chapter 9. In such a trial, many subjects are randomly assigned to receive either an investigational new drug, a placebo, or an established therapy if one exists. Neither the treating doctors nor the patients know which they are receiving. All patients are monitored for adverse events and responses to treatment. Hoped-for outcomes must be defined before the study begins to avoid identifying apparently effective results after the study ends. At the end of the study, investigators disclose which individuals received the new drug and which did not. Adverse events and responses to treatment are then compared between the two groups. A rigorous statistical analysis must be performed to establish with the highest degree of probability that any detected differences are real and not merely a result of chance. Results from studies such as these are what the FDA usually requires before approving a drug. To the best of my knowledge, there are *no* randomized, double-blind, placebo-controlled studies for any alternative treatments of chronic hepatitis C; therefore, their safety and effectiveness have not been scientifically proven.

In the world of alternative medicine, silymarin, which is present in milk thistle, has become the preferred substance to help anyone and everyone with a liver disease. Some individuals even advocate taking it to keep the liver healthy. But there is no scientific evidence that silymarin or milk thistle is an effective treatment or preventive agent for any liver disease. At present, I am aware of one study subjecting silymarin to a randomized, double-blind clinical trial. Until this trial determines whether silymarin is safe or effective for patients with chronic hepatitis C, it should be considered an experimental therapy that could be potentially dangerous. Patients should *not* take these substances except as part of an Insititutional Review Board–approved clinical trial.

What about apparently safe alternative therapies that do not involve ingestion of substances or dangerous manipulations, such as music and massage therapy? Patients who use these alternative therapies are not putting their lives in danger as users of unapproved herbs or drugs may be. My opinion is that patients should consider these measures as complementary but absolutely *not* as substitutes for medical care. Such therapies will not cure chronic hepatitis C; however, they may help a patient feel better in other ways, such as relaxing tense patients.

Many proponents of alternative medicine believe that there is a healthy liver diet or healthy liver lifestyle for patients with chronic hepatitis C, as well as for all people. Many alternative or holistic products include preparations for a healthy liver, heart, or kidneys. There are *no* special substances or diets for a healthy liver. A lifestyle that is conducive to general good health is good for the liver. All individuals should minimize fat in their diets and maintain an ideal weight by watching what they eat and by regular exercise. This will avoid the accumulation of fat in the liver, just as it will in all other parts of the body. Common sense should be used when it comes to drinking. Alcohol consumption in moderation will not hurt the liver, but excessive drinking can. Other substances or activities that can damage the liver should also be avoided, such as injection of illicit drugs, as well as drugs, herbs, and remedies that may be toxic.

In many cases, alternative therapies for chronic hepatitis C will be safe but of no value. They can, however, be detrimental. Before trying anything for chronic hepatitis C, consult your doctor. *Always beware of unscrupulous purveyors of unproved remedies!*

Appendix

References and Other Sources of Information

MANY PATIENTS WANT to know more about hepatitis C. They want up-to-date information that goes far beyond this book. Where should they look?

Newspapers such as the *New York Times* or the *Wall Street Journal* will frequently report major findings related to hepatitis C. Information related to new drugs that influence pharmaceutical companies will often be reported in the business sections of major newspapers. Major television news organizations and even local news stations will usually report major breakthroughs. The Internet is another source; however, one must keep in mind its dangers, in particular the proliferation of disease-related Web sites not monitored by health professionals.

For laypersons who want to learn about hepatitis C in depth, or to keep up with the most current literature, I have provided some references and sources where you can find more information. Please note that these lists are not complete but rather my personal recommendations of what I think are the most useful.

Medical Textbooks Aimed at Health Professionals

Most doctors start with a textbook when looking for more information on a disease or condition. Remember, no textbook is absolutely authoritative and some are better than others in different areas. *Textbooks also become outdated.* The information in even the most current medical textbooks is usually at least a year old or older. Finally, textbooks are not gospel and some of their facts may be wrong.

There are numerous textbooks devoted to internal medicine and pediatrics. Others are specifically focused on liver diseases. The best source for these textbooks is a medical school library. They are most likely to be up-to-date. These books are very expensive and I do not recommend buying one unless you are a physician or medical student. Some of the most widely used textbooks of liver disease are listed below. These are frequently updated and newer editions will usually be available from year to year.

Bircher, J., ed. *Oxford Textbook of Clinical Hepatology,* 2d ed. Oxford University Press, 1999.

Schiff, E. R., M. F. Sorrell, and W. C. Maddrey, eds. *Schiff's Diseases of the Liver,* 8th ed. Lippincott, Williams & Wilkins Publishers, 1998.

Sherlock, S., and J. Dooley, contributors. *Diseases of the Liver and Biliary System,* 10th ed. Blackwell Science, Inc., 1997.

Zakim, D., and T. D. Boyer, eds. *Hepatology: A Textbook of Liver Disease,* 3d ed. W. B. Saunders Co., 1996.

Medical and Scientific Journals

Discoveries that will ultimately be important in understanding liver diseases may be published in highly technical journals. These papers are usually incomprehensible to the nonspecialist (and even most practicing physicians). However, some scientific journals publish papers that have an immediate impact on clinical liver disease, such as the discovery of the hepatitis C virus in 1989.

The most significant clinical papers on hepatitis C are usually published in the most important general medical journals. Several specialized journals, such as *Hepatology*, the official journal of the American Association for the Study of Liver Diseases, publish papers on both clinical hepatology and basic science related to liver diseases. Some of the medical journals most likely to have important papers on hepatitis C are listed below. You can also search the up-to-date medical literature by using Pub Med on the Internet (www.ncbi.nlm.nih.gov), available through the National Center for Biotechnology Information. Pub Med contains a text search engine and provides references for articles and abstracts from many of them.

Predominantly Basic Scientific Journals

Cell (a premier general scientific journal)
Current Biology (an excellent general scientific journal)
Immunity (immune system)
Journal of Biological Chemistry (basic biochemistry of virus)
Journal of Cell Biology (cell biology of viruses)
Journal of Cell Science (cell biology of viruses)
Journal of Clinical Investigation (general biomedicine)
Journal of Experimental Medicine (immune system and some virology)
Journal of General Virology (devoted to the study of viruses)
Journal of Immunology (immune system)
Journal of Virology (probably best journal devoted to the study of viruses)
Molecular and Cellular Biology (molecular biology and virology)
Nature (a premier general scientific journal)
Nature Biotechnology (biotechnology breakthroughs)
Nature Genetics (genetic basis of diseases)
Nature Medicine (general biomedicine)
Nature Structural Biology (structure of macromolecules)

Proceedings of the National Academy of Sciences USA (excellent general scientific journal)
Science (a premier general scientific journal)
Structure (structure of macromolecules)
Virology (devoted to the study of viruses)

Leading General Medical Journals

Annals of Internal Medicine
Lancet
New England Journal of Medicine

Medical Journals Focused on Liver Diseases (Science and Clinical)

American Journal of Gastroenterology
Gastroenterology
Gut
Hepato-gastroenterology
Hepatology
Journal of Hepatology
Journal of Viral Hepatitis (specialized in viral hepatitis)
Liver

Reputable Internet Resources

Many patients and their friends and family members are turning to the Internet for medical information and even advice. In the past few years, there has been an incredible proliferation of medical Web sites. Some are excellent and some are frankly dangerous, professing miracle cures and knowledge that they claim doctors and scientists do not know about. In using the Internet, *be careful.* Anyone can put up an impressive-looking Web site and make ridiculous or misleading information look important. People can masquerade as doctors and professors and provide medical advice. *Never accept*

*medical advice from anyone except a doctor who has taken your
complete medical history and examined you.*

The Web sites I recommend that provide information on hepatitis C are given below There are thousands of medical Web sites, many of which also have information on hepatitis C. I have not listed general medical Web sites, only those specifically devoted to liver diseases and hepatitis C. This list is not comprehensive; I apologize for any reputable Web sites I have omitted.

American Association for the Study of Liver Diseases
www.aasld.org
*Homepage of the predominant American organization for
physicians and biomedical scientists with an interest in
the liver and its diseases.*

American Liver Foundation
www.liverfoundation.org
*The American Liver Foundation is a national, voluntary
health agency dedicated to preventing, treating, and
curing hepatitis and all liver diseases.*

Diseases of the Liver
cpmcnet.columbia.edu/dept/gi/disliv.html
My own site at Columbia University.

Hepatitis Branch Homepage Centers for Disease Control
and Prevention
www.cdc.gov/ncidod/diseases/hepatitis/index.htm
*The homepage of the Hepatitis Branch of the Centers for
Disease Control and Prevention, the government organization
whose mission is the control of infectious diseases.*

HepNet
www.hepnet.com
*A comprehensive site with lots of excellent information
on viral hepatitis. Although not strictly a company site, I
should point out that the person who created and*

maintains this site is an employee of Schering-Plough, a company that has a financial interest in selling drugs to treat hepatitis C.

National Center for Biotechnology Information
www.ncbi.nlm.nih.gov
This Web site provides the user with access to Pub Med to search the primary medical literature. Abstracts are available for many articles. It also contains a fantastic collection of biomedical resources, including DNA sequence information and the results of the publicly funded Human Genome Project.

National Institute of Diabetes and Digestive and Kidney Diseases (NIDDK)
www.niddk.nih.gov
NIDDK is an institute of the U.S. National Institutes of Health, devoted to most issues regarding digestive diseases.

Glossary

THE MEDICAL TERMINOLOGY used by doctors can be difficult to understand. New jargon has developed over the years that is unique to hepatitis C. This glossary defines some of the medical terms relevant to liver disease and hepatitis C.

Activity A unit of measurement used by biochemists that is proportional to the amount of an enzyme at a given temperature, concentration, and other conditions. Various blood tests used to assess patients with liver disorders, such as aminotransferases, are reported in units of activity per volume of blood.

Albumin The most abundant protein in the blood, synthesized in the liver. Its concentration in the blood may be low when liver function is compromised.

Alcoholic A person with either an alcohol abuse or alcohol dependency disorder. These disorders are defined clinically in the American Psychiatric Association's *Diagnostic and Statistical Manual of Mental Disorders*.

Alkaline phosphatase An enzyme present in the bile ducts, as well as bones, kidneys, and placenta. Its activity is frequently measured in the blood and elevations may indicate bile duct or liver disease.

ALT An abbreviation for alanine aminotransferase, an enzyme present in hepatocytes (the predominant liver cell type) that leaks out of cells if they are damaged or die. The activity of ALT activity per unit of blood is measured in the clinical laboratory and is often elevated in hepatitis.

Aminotransferases Enzymes present in hepatocytes (and other tissues). The activities of two aminotransferases, alanine aminotransferase (ALT) and aspartate aminotransferase (AST), are frequently measured in the blood. These enzymes leak out of hepatocytes if they are damaged or die. Their blood activities are often elevated in liver diseases such as hepatitis.

Antibodies Proteins in the blood produced by cells of the immune system, which can recognize components of infecting organisms such as viruses or bacteria. Individuals chronically infected with the hepatitis C virus usually develop antibodies against the virus that are detected in diagnostic tests for infection.

Antigen A protein or other type of chemical compound recognized by an antibody. *See also* Antibodies.

Ascites Abnormal accumulation of edema fluid in the abdomen. *See also* Edema.

AST An abbreviation for aspartate aminotransferase, an enzyme present in hepatocytes (the predominant liver cell type) and other tissue, particularly muscle, that leaks out of cells if they are damaged or die. The activity of AST activity per unit of blood is measured in the clinical laboratory and is often elevated in hepatitis.

bDNA A type of blood test sometimes used to measure the amount of hepatitis C viral RNA in the blood.

Bilirubin A chemical compound that is produced in the human body primarily from the breakdown of old red blood cells. It is taken up by the liver, changed to a more soluble form, and then secreted into the bile. The blood bilirubin concentration is often measured in the clinical laboratory and may be elevated in various liver diseases, as well as in some conditions in which red blood cells are destroyed at an abnormal rate. If the blood bilirubin concentration is higher than about 2 milligrams per deciliter, the person will appear jaundiced.

Breakthrough An individual with chronic hepatitis C treated with an interferon alpha-based therapy who initially does not have detectable hepatitis C viral RNA in his or her blood during treatment but which becomes detectable later in the course of treatment.

Bridging fibrosis A type of scarring seen in liver biopsies, which indicates a high probability that the liver will develop cirrhosis.

Cachexia A generalized wasting, especially of muscle mass, which can be seen in advanced cirrhosis as well as other chronic diseases.

CAT scan Computerized axial tomography; an x-ray test used to obtain cross-sectional images of the body. It may be useful in evaluation of the liver and gallbladder, especially in searching for tumors, gallstones, or evidence of bile duct obstruction. It does not provide useful information about the degree of fibrosis or inflammation in chronic hepatitis.

Cholestasis Stagnation of bile flow in the liver.

Cirrhosis Fibrosis (scarring) and widespread nodules in the liver. It can result from many years of chronic hepatitis C as well as any chronic liver disease.

Clinical trial An experimental protocol in which a new drug, new way of giving a drug, or an old drug for a new indication is tested. Often divided into Phase I, which establishes safety; Phase II, which tests for some efficacy and obtains more data on safety; and Phase III, which establishes efficacy and safety compared to a placebo (dummy drug) or another therapy.

Conjugation The chemical reaction in bilirubin metabolism in which glucuronic acid moieties are coupled to bilirubin to make it soluble so that it can be secreted into the bile.

Conjugation takes place in the hepatocytes of the liver and is catalyzed by the enzyme UDP-glucuronosyltransferase. Other substances, such as drugs and toxins, may also be conjugated in the liver to make them more soluble for elimination in either the bile or by the kidneys.

Control group In a clinical trial, the group of subjects who receives a placebo or an already approved therapy.

Cryoglobulinemina The condition defined by the presence of cryoglobulins in the blood. *See also* Cryoglobulins.

Cryoglobulins Protein complexes that circulate in the blood and precipitate out at cold temperatures. In chronic hepatitis C, cryoglobulins are probably a combination of viral components and certain antibodies against the virus. Cryoglobulins can deposit in the kidneys and cause them to malfunction.

CT scan *See* CAT scan.

Deoxyribonucleic acid (DNA) The genetic material of animals and plants.

Edema Abnormal accumulation of fluids in the tissues of the body. It can occur in advanced cirrhosis.

Encephalopathy Abnormal mental functioning secondary to organic causes. *See also* Hepatic encephalopathy.

Endoscope A fiber-optic tube used to visualize the inside of body cavities, including the upper and lower gastrointestinal tract. In patients with liver diseases, endoscopy may be necessary to visualize the esophagus, stomach, or proximal small intestine. These tubes may be modified so that procedures can be performed through them under direct visualization.

Endoscopic retrograde cholangiopancreatography (ERCP) A procedure in which a small tube is inserted into the bile duct via an endoscope and dye is injected. An x-ray image of the bile ducts inside and outside the liver as well as the ducts of the pancreas can then be obtained, because x-rays cannot pass through the injected dye. The action can be modified to do other procedures such as remove gallstones trapped in a large bile duct or place a drainage tube into the duct.

Endoscopic rubber band ligation A procedure in which esophageal, or possibly gastric, varices are tied off through a fiber-optic tube (endoscope) under direct visualization.

Endoscopic sclerotherapy A procedure in which esophageal varices are treated with a caustic chemical to occlude them. This procedure is performed under direct visualization via a fiber-optic tube (endoscope).

Enlarged liver *See* Hepatomegaly.

Envelope A fatty structure that surrounds the hepatitis C viral particle.

Enzyme A protein that catalyzes (speeds up) a chemical reaction.

ERCP *See* Endoscopic retrograde cholangiopancreatography.

Esophageal varices Varicose veins in the esophagus, which can occur in cirrhosis. They can rupture and cause life-threatening internal bleeding.

FDA Food and Drug Administration; the U.S. federal government agency that approves and regulates the use of drugs, with particular emphasis on safety and clinical efficacy.

Fibrosis Scar tissue that can develop in the liver in patients with chronic hepatitis C.

Gamma-glutamyltranspeptidase Often abbreviated as GGTP, it is an enzyme present in the bile ducts. Its activity in the blood is frequently measured in the clinical laboratory. Elevations can indicate a wide variety of liver diseases and may be high in some individuals without any significant disease. It may be elevated in patients who consume excessive alcohol or who are taking certain drugs. It may also indicate bile duct disease.

Gastric varices Varicose veins in the stomach, which can occur in cirrhosis. They can rupture and cause life-threatening internal bleeding.

Gastroenterologist A doctor who specializes in diseases of the digestive system, including the liver. Some gastroenterologists, however, prefer to care primarily for patients with diseases of the esophagus, stomach, intestines, and rectum and do not devote much time to liver diseases.

Genome The total genetic material of an organism.

Genotypes Slightly different strains of the hepatitis C virus, classified based on the sequences of their genetic material. The hepatitis C virus is generally divided into six different genotypes and several subtypes. Genotype 1 responds less well to interferon alpha-based treatments.

GGTP *See* Gamma-glutamyltranspeptidase.

Grade A numerical score given to indicate the degree of inflammation seen in a liver biopsy.

Gynecomastia Breast enlargement in men that can occur as a result of cirrhosis and poor metabolism of circulating estrogens in the blood.

Half-life When referring to a drug, the amount of time it takes for one half of the dose to be eliminated from the body.

HCV An abbreviation often used for hepatitis C.

Helicase An enzyme that unwinds DNA (DNA helicase) or RNA (RNA helicase). The hepatitis C virus encodes an RNA helicase that unwinds its RNA. Drugs are under development to inhibit this enzyme.

Helicase inhibitor A drug that inhibits a helicase. *See also* Helicase.

Hep C An abbreviation often used for hepatitis C.

Hepatic artery A blood vessel that delivers oxygen-rich blood to the liver directly from the heart.

Hepatic encephalopathy A change in mental state caused by the inability of the liver to metabolize ammonia and other nitrogen-containing toxins that are absorbed from the gut and are toxic to the brain; can range from subtle changes in the ability to concentrate to deep coma.

Hepatic vein The major vein via which blood exits the liver.

Hepatitis Inflammation of the liver. There are many causes of hepatitis, including alcohol, drugs, toxins, viruses, and metabolic disorders. Infection with the hepatitis C virus is one of these causes.

Hepatocellular carcinoma A primary liver cancer.

Hepatocyte The primary cell type of the liver. Many different biochemical reactions essential for whole-body metabolism and health take place in hepatocytes.

Hepatologist A doctor who specializes in diseases of the liver.

Hepatology The study of liver diseases.

Hepatomegaly Enlarged liver. There are many causes, including some diseases of the liver.

Hepatorenal syndrome A type of kidney failure that is seen only in patients with liver failure. It is virtually always fatal unless liver transplantation is performed.

Hyperbilirubinemia Elevated bilirubin concentration in the blood.

Hypoalbuminemia Low albumin concentration in the blood.

Immunosuppressive drugs A class of drugs used to suppress the immune system and prevent organ transplant rejection. Some are also used to treat autoimmune hepatitis.

Inflammation A physiological response characterized by the infiltration of tissue with certain types of white blood cells.

Interferon Naturally occurring proteins that have many functions in the body, including helping to fight off viral infections. Synthetic types of interferon, administered by injection, are used in the treatment of hepatitis C. They are also used for the treatment of hepatitis B, some cancers, and multiple sclerosis.

Interferon alpha The type of interferon used to treat chronic hepatitis C, hepatitis B, and some cancers.

Jaundice Yellowing of the skin, whites of the eyes, and mucous membranes secondary to high bilirubin concentrations in the blood.

Liver biopsy A procedure in which a small piece of liver tissue is obtained to examine under the microscope. It is usually done with a needle through the skin but can be done at surgery or via other approaches.

Liver enzymes Various blood tests that are related to the liver. Generally used to refer to the aminotransferases (ALT and AST); also used to refer to alkaline phosphatase and gamma-glutamyltranspeptidase.

Liver function tests A term inappropriately and unfortunately frequently used for various blood tests related to the liver. Generally used to refer to the aminotransferases (ALT and AST), it may also be used to refer to alkaline phosphatase and gamma-glutamyltranspeptidase. This term should *not* be used, as these blood tests do not assess liver function.

Liver palms Reddish palms (palmar erythema), which may be seen in individuals with various liver diseases.

Liver–spleen scan A nuclear medicine test that can sometimes detect cirrhosis.

Long-term responder *See* Sustained responder.

Milk thistle *See* Silymarin.

MRI scan Magnetic resonance imaging; an imaging study of the part of the body that uses the phenomenon known as nuclear magnetic resonance. It is sometimes used to visualize the liver and may be useful in searching for certain types of tumors. It does not provide useful information about the degree of fibrosis or inflammation in chronic hepatitis.

Naive An individual with chronic hepatitis C who has not been treated for the disease.

Nonresponder A patient with chronic hepatitis C who is treated with interferon alpha-based therapy but continues to have detectable viral RNA in his or her blood during treatment.

Nonstructural proteins Proteins of the hepatitis C virus that are not components of the viral particle but are expressed in infected cells and essential for viral replication.

Paracentesis A procedure in which fluid (ascites) is removed from the abdominal cavity by inserting a needle through the abdominal wall. A small amount of fluid may be removed for diagnostic purposes or a large amount for therapeutic reasons.

PCR *See* Polymerase chain reaction.

PEG An abbreviation for polyethylene glycol, an inert compound that is attached to interferon alpha to prolong its half-life in the body.

Peginterferon Interferon attached to polyethylene glycol. Peginterferons have longer half-lives in the body than unmodified interferon.

Pegylated A protein with polyethylene glycol attached (for example, pegylated interferon).

Pegylation The chemical process by which polyethylene glycol is added to a protein.

Platelets The smallest blood cells that play a role in blood clotting. The platelet count is sometimes low in people with cirrhosis.

Polyethylene glycol An inert compound that is attached to interferon alpha to prolong its half-life in the body. Polyethylene glycol is also used as antifreeze in car radiators.

Polymerase An enzyme that catalyzes reactions in which certain molecules are made longer. Some types of DNA polymerase are used in the polymerase chain reaction to detect hepatitis C virus genetic material in the blood. The hepatitis C virus contains an RNA-directed RNA polymer ase that catalyzes the replication of its RNA genome.

Polymerase chain reaction (PCR) A type of chemical reaction used to amplify small amounts of DNA of a specific sequence. This type of chemical reaction, combined with reverse transcription or copying of RNA to DNA, is used to detect hepatitis C virus RNA in the blood.

Portal gastropathy Diffusely dilated veins in the stomach that result from portal hypertension.

Portal hypertension High pressure in the portal vein and connected veins, usually caused by cirrhosis. Portal hypertension can lead to many problems, including the development of gastric and esophageal varices and splenomegaly.

Portal vein The major blood vessel that supplies blood to the liver. Blood in the portal vein contains substances absorbed from the stomach and gut.

Protease An enzyme that catalyzes the cutting of a protein. The hepatitis C virus encodes two proteases that cut viral proteins and are essential for viral reproduction. Drugs targeted against the hepatitis C virus proteases, generically known as protease inhibitors, are being developed.

Protease inhibitor A drug that inhibits a protease. *See also* Protease.

Prothrombin time A blood test used to measure the amounts of certain clotting factors in the blood. It may be prolonged if liver function is abnormal. It may also be prolonged in other disorders.

Pruritus Itching; a symptom of some liver diseases, including hepatitis C.

Quasispecies Slightly different variants of the hepatitis C virus that arise by mutations in the viral RNA.

Red blood cells Cells that circulate in the blood, whose function is to carry oxygen.

Relapser A patient with chronic hepatitis C who does not have detectable hepatitis C viral RNA in his or her blood during treatment with an interferon alpha-based therapy, but again has detectable viral RNA after stopping treatment.

Responder A patient with chronic hepatitis C who does not have detectable hepatitis C viral RNA in his or her blood during or after treatment.

Ribavirin An orally administered drug used in combination with interferon alpha in the treatment of chronic hepatitis C.

Ribonucleic acid (RNA) The genetic material of the hepatitis C virus. Animal and plant cells use RNA for different purposes, primarily for translating DNA into protein.

RNA helicase *See* Helicase.

RNA polymerase An enzyme that makes RNA molecules longer. The hepatitis C virus contains an RNA-directed RNA polymerase that catalyzes the copying of its RNA genome and is essential for viral replication. Drugs that inhibit the RNA polymerase of the hepatitis C virus are currently under development.

RNA polymerase inhibitor A drug that inhibits an RNA polymerase. *See also* RNA polymerase.

Shunt A surgical procedure in which a vein of the portal circulation is connected to a blood vein of the systemic circulation to relieve portal hypertension. Radiologists also use a type of shunt. *See also* Transjugular intrahepatic portosystemic shunt.

Silymarin A compound found in milk thistle championed by followers of alternative or herbal medicine as a treatment for many liver disorders, including chronic hepatitis C. It has not been shown to be effective or even safe for use by patients with liver diseases.

Sonogram *See* Ultrasound.

Spenomegaly An enlarged spleen that can be caused by portal hypertension.

Spider angiomata Small red marks on the skin with "legs" that radiate out from the center, making them look like spiders. If pressure is applied, they blanch and then turn red again when pressure is released. They are seen in patients with chronic liver diseases and sometimes in pregnant women.

Stage A numerical score given to indicate the degree of fibrosis seen on a liver biopsy.

Steatosis Fatty liver.

Structural proteins Hepatitis C viral proteins that are part of the mature viral particle. They include the core protein and two envelope proteins.

Sustained responder A patient with chronic hepatitis C who does not have detectable hepatitis C viral RNA in his or her blood six months or longer after a course of treatment.

Thrombocytopenia Low platelet count.

Transjugular intrahepatic portosystemic shunt (TIPS) A procedure performed by radiologists in which a tube is passed through the liver to connect the portal and hepatic veins and reduce portal hypertension. It is indicated to stop bleeding from gastric and esophageal varices.

Ultrasound An imaging study that uses sound waves to obtain an image of internal organs. Often used to image the liver and gallbladder, it is an excellent test to look for liver tumors, gallstones, and bile duct obstruction. It does not provide useful information about the degree of fibrosis or inflammation in chronic hepatitis.

Vena cava The largest vein of the body that returns blood to the heart. The hepatic vein, through which blood exits the liver, empties directly into the vena cava.

About the Author

HOWARD J. WORMAN, M.D., is Associate Professor of Medicine and Anatomy and Cell Biology at the College of Physicians and Surgeons of Columbia University. He is also Associate Attending Physician and Director of the Division of Digestive and Liver Diseases of the Medical Service of the New York–Presbyterian Hospital Columbia-Presbyterian Center. Dr. Worman received an A.B. cum laude in biology and chemistry from Cornell University and an M.D. from the University of Chicago. He did residency training in internal medicine at New York Hospital and postdoctoral research in Cell Biology in the laboratory of Nobel Laureate Dr. Günter Blobel at Rockefeller University. After a stint as an Assistant Professor at the Mount Sinai School of Medicine, where he obtained clinical training in liver diseases, Dr. Worman moved to Columbia University. Dr. Worman is an author of numerous medical and scientific papers, creator of the "Diseases of the Liver" World Wide Web site (cpmcnet.columbia.edu/dept/gi/disliv.html), and author of *The Liver Disorders Sourcebook*. His laboratory research is focused on basic cell biology, hepatitis C virus infection, and autoimmune liver diseases. His clinical research is focused on the treatment of chronic hepatitis C and other liver diseases.

Index